Antibiotics and Chemotherapy

Current Topics

Antibiotics and Chemotherapy

Current Topics

Edited by

R. N. Grüneberg

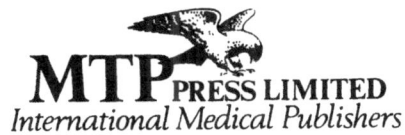

MTPPRESS LIMITED
International Medical Publishers

Published by
MTP Press Limited
Falcon House
Lancaster, England

Copyright © 1980 MTP Press Limited
Softcover reprint of the hardcover 1st edition 1980

First published 1980

British Library Cataloguing in Publication Data

Antibiotics and chemotherapy: current topics –
(Current status of modern therapy; vol. 4)

1. Antibiotics
I. Gruneberg, R N II. Series
615'.329   RM267

ISBN 978-94-011-7196-0   ISBN 978-94-011-7194-6 (eBook)
DOI 10.1007/978-94-011-7194-6
Phototypesetting by Swiftpages Limited, Liverpool
and printed by
Clarke-Constable Ltd, Edinburgh

Contents

List of Contributors

M. W. CASEWELL, BSc, MD, MRCPath
Senior Lecturer and Honorary Consultant Microbiologist, St
Thomas' Hospital, London, SE1 7EH

R. N. GRÜNEBERG, MD, MRCPath
Consultant Microbiologist, University College Hospital, London,
WC1E 6AU

M. N. LOGAN, MB ChB
Department of Medical Microbiology, Dudley Road Hospital,
Birmingham, B18 7QH

G. L. RIDGWAY, MD, BSc, MRCPath
Consultant Microbiologist, University College Hospital, London,
WC1E 6AU

J. B. SELKON, TD, MB Ch B, FRCPath, DCP
Director, Regional Public Health Laboratory, Newcastle General
Hospital, Newcastle-upon-Tyne, NE4 6BE

D. C. SHANSON, MB, MRCS, MRCPath
Consultant Microbiologist, St Stephen's Hospital, Chelsea, Lon-
don, SW10 9TH, and Senior Lecturer in Medical Microbiology,
Westminster Hospital Medical School, London, SW1P 2AR

N. A. SIMMONS, MD, MRCS, FRCPath
Consultant Clinical Microbiologist, Guy's Hospital, London, SE1
9RT

vii

J. D. WILLIAMS, BSc, MD, MRCPath
Professor of Medical Microbiology, The London Hospital Medical College, London, E1 2AD

R. J. WILLIAMS, BSc, PhD
Lecturer in Medical Microbiology, The London Hospital Medical College, London, E1 2AD

R. WISE, MRCPath
Department of Medical Microbiology, Dudley Road Hospital, Birmingham, B18 7QH

Consultant Editor's Note

Current Status of Modern Therapy

Series Editor: J. Marks, Girton College, Cambridge

The *Current Status of Modern Therapy* is a major new series from MTP Press with the purpose of providing a definitive view of modern therapeutic practice in those areas of clinical medicine in which important changes are occurring. The series consists of monographs specially commissioned under the individual editorship of internationally recognized experts in their fields. Their selection of a panel of contributors from many countries ensures an international perspective on developments in therapy.

The series will aim to review the growth areas of clinical pharmacology and therapeutics in a systematic way. It will be a continuing series in which the same subject areas will be covered by revised editions as advances make this desirable.

The literature on antibiotics and chemotherapy is very extensive and it could be held adequately covers the field. A search however shows that advances are still being made in this research area.

Dr Grüneberg who has worked and published extensively on antibacterial therapy has followed the guidelines for the series excellently in the selection of topics and authors for this fourth volume in the series: *Antibiotics and Chemotherapy*. He has selected the interesting growth areas and contentious topics and then invited acknowledged experts to present their views. The volume will I am sure be widely valued for its practical approach to these problems.

Preface

The purpose of this book is to provide reviews of various antibiotic topics which will be of interest to practising clinicians and to microbiologists. It is hoped that enough references have been provided to enable the enthusiast to immerse himself in the source literature.

No attempt has been made to cover the whole field, which is well catered for in the numerous works on the subject. Rather, the intention has been to select a number of topics in which there has been a great deal of change in recent years, and to ask an appropriate authority to review the subject. Since I chose the topics, it may be supposed, quite correctly, that I have identified subjects in which I felt myself to require some postgraduate education. The process was something like the well known radio programme in which a castaway is allowed to select a number of gramophone records to take with him to a desert island. I hope that readers will share my interest in the contributions from a number of distinguished contributors to the field of antibiotic chemotherapeutic research.

Although I have had the privilege of editing this volume it will be understood that the views expressed by the authors are their own and have not been the subject of editorial review. I am grateful to all the collaborators in this volume, and to the publishers, MTP Press, for their help, and for asking me to undertake the task.

R. N. GRÜNEBERG

1

The chemotherapy of infective endocarditis

D. C. Shanson

INTRODUCTION

The incidence of infective endocarditis in recent years is similar to that noted in 1939[1]. The overall mortality has fallen from 100% before the age of chemotherapy to about 30% 30 years ago but has not been further reduced[1,2].

The pattern of the disease has significantly changed during the last 30 years in respect of the ages of the patients, the causative organisms, the predisposing factors and the clinical modes of presentation[1-3]. In particular (a) the disease affects more elderly patients than in the past, with a preponderance of patients over the age of 50 years; (b) there is a wider range of causative organisms than before and a somewhat decreased incidence of cases where alpha-haemolytic viridans streptococci are the causative organisms; (c) rheumatic heart disease is less important than in the past but congenital heart disease is more important; (d) other important predisposing factors now include cardiac surgery to insert prosthetic valves, drug addiction and aortic atherosclerotic valve disease; (e) pyrexia, heart murmurs and cardiac failure are still important clinical features but in many more patients than previously the symptoms are minimal at the time of first presentation.

A rational approach to the chemotherapy of infective endocarditis is dependent on a knowledge of the current aetiology of the disease. At all stages in the management of patients with suspected endocarditis, there should be the closest collaboration between the clinician and microbiologist.

1

AETIOLOGY

Bacteria (over 100 different species), fungi, the rickettsia-like organism *Coxiella burnetti* and *Chlamydia psittaci* may cause infective endocarditis. The most frequently occurring causative organisms in endocarditis patients who have not had previous heart surgery are included in Table 1, in patients who have had previous heart surgery in Table 2, and in patients who are main line drug addicts in Table 3.

Table 1   Some organisms causing endocarditis in patients who have not had heart surgery

Organism	Positive blood culture cases (%)	Author references
Streptococci		
'Streptococcus viridans'	44–73	2, 33, 111, 117, 118
Streptococcus faecalis	7–18	2, 27, 40
β-haemolytic streptococcus	7	2
Anaerobic streptococcus		2
Staphylococci		
Staphylococcus aureus	9–17	2, 24, 119
Staphylococcus epidermidis	0–5	2, 33
Haemophilus spp.		
Haemophilus influenzae		
Haemophilus parainfluenzae	1–3	19, 54, 70, 120
Haemophilus aphrophilus		

Streptococci

Over 30 years ago '*Streptococcus viridans*' caused more than 85% of cases of endocarditis which mainly occurred in adults less than 40 years of age with rheumatic heart disease[4]. Although viridans streptococci cause endocarditis less frequently than in the past they are still the most common cause of endocarditis (Table 1). Most cases of endocarditis in patients who have had previous heart surgery are of late onset and in

Table 2 Some organisms causing endocarditis in patients with prosthetic heart valves

Organism	Confirmed endocarditis cases(%)		Author references
	Early onset*	Late onset†	
Streptococci			
'Streptococcus viridans'	0–5	27–41 ⎤	
			19, 69
Streptococcus faecalis	0–6	0–10 ⎦	
Staphylococci and diphtheroids			
Staphylococcus aureus	17–44	10–13 ⎤	
			19, 69, 121
Staphylococcus epidermidis	6–25	3–23 ⎦	
Diphtheroids	6–12	3	19, 69
Gram-negative bacilli			
Gram-negative bacilli including:			
Klebsiella, Proteus, Enterobacter, ⎤			
Pseudomonas, Serratia spp. and ⎬ 17–37		8–31	
E. coli ⎦			
Fungi			
Candida spp.	17	4 ⎤	
			19
Aspergillus spp.	2	2 ⎦	

* Within 2 months of cardiac surgery
† Majority of cases of prosthetic valve endocarditis occur at least 2 months after cardiac surgery

these patients viridans streptococci are also the most frequent cause of endocarditis (Table 2).

Recently only about 50% of medical endocarditis cases were stated to be due to viridans streptococci[5] whereas another author has given a figure of 80%[6]. Difficulties arise because various non-haemolytic and microaerophilic streptococci are included as 'Streptococcus viridans' by one author while another author only includes alpha-haemolytic streptococci in this term. Different interpretations of the term 'Streptococcus viridans' by various authorities are summarised in Table 4. This term now represents many different species of streptococci that normally occur in the mouth. Parker and Ball have shown that there is a close

Table 3 Some organisms causing endocarditis in drug addicts[122–127]

Organism†	Confirmed endocarditis cases(%)*
Staphylococci	
Staphylococcus aureus	Approx 60%
Staphylococcus epidermidis	Less than 3%
Gram-negative bacilli	
Gram-negative bacilli including:	
mainly *Klebsiella, Enterobacter,* *E. coli* and *Pseudomonas* organisms	Approx. 20%
Streptococci	
Streptococci including haemolytic strepto- cocci and enterococci	Approx. 10%
Fungi *Candida* spp.	Approx. 10%

† Frequently multi-microbial endocarditis occurs in addicts
* Author references 122–127

association between *Streptococcus sanguis, mitior* and *mutans* with endocarditis[7]. These authors also showed that *Streptococcus bovis* was an important streptococcal cause of endocarditis. This organism, like *Streptococcus mutans*, is usually non-haemolytic and sensitive to penicillin. *Streptococcus bovis* is a Lancefield group D streptococcus that has previously been confused with *Streptococcus faecalis*. From the chemotherapeutic point of view it is appropriate to regard *Streptococcus bovis* as a viridans streptococcus. Authors who separate non-haemolytic and microaerophilic streptococci from '*Streptococcus viridans*' and the enterococci will get different percentages for the causative organisms of endocarditis from those using a modern classification of streptococci.

The author's suggestions for a simple streptococcal classification of relevance from a chemotherapeutic aspect are given in Table 5. The full identification of alpha- or non-haemolytic streptococci, other than *Streptococcus faecalis*, is usually of little importance to those giving advice about immediate chemotherapy.

Table 4 What is meant by 'Streptococcus viridans'?

Bacteria included as 'Streptococcus viridans'	Characteristic haemolysis on blood agar		Author references
	Alpha-	Non-	
(A) Alpha-haemolytic streptococci (resistant to Optochin)	+		128
(B)			
i) Streptococcus sanguis	+		
ii) Streptococcus mitior	+		
iii) Streptococcus mutans		+	129, 130
iv) Streptococcus Milleri		+	
v) Streptococcus salivarius		+	

Table 5   A simple classification of streptococci to aid the chemotherapy of endocarditis

Organism	Usual haemolysis	Antimicrobial sensitivity to penicillin
(A) 'Streptococcus viridans'		
Streptococcus sanguis	Alpha-	
Streptococcus mitior	Alpha-	
Streptococcus mutans Streptococcus milleri	Non- Non-	Usually highly sensitive, (MIC equal to or less than 0.12 mg/l) – penicillin alone usually bactericidal
Streptococcus bovis	Non-	
Miscellaneous alpha-haemolytic streptococci*	Alpha-	
Miscellaneous non-haemolytic streptococci†	Non-	
(B) 'Streptococcus faecalis'		
Streptococcus faecalis Streptococcus faecium	Non- Non-	Usually lower sensitivity – combination of penicillin with aminoglycoside necessary for a total bactericidal effect
(C) Beta-haemolytic streptococci		
Streptococcus pyogenes Group B haemolytic streptococcus	Beta Beta	Highly sensitive to penicillin. Lower sensitivity to penicillin with aminoglycoside may be necessary for bactericidal effect – combination
(D) Anaerobic streptococci		
Peptococcus and pepto streptococcus		Variable sensitivity to penicillin – consider penicillin plus metronidazole

* excluding pneumococci
† excluding *Streptococcus faecalis*

Staphylococci
After streptococci, staphylococci are the next most frequent cause of endocarditis (Tables 1 and 2). *Staphylococcus aureus* (coagulase positive) is the main cause in drug addicts (Table 3).

In patients with prosthetic valves both *Staphylococcus aureus* and *Staphylococcus epidermidis* are important causes of endocarditis. Most strains of both these species are resistant to penicillin.

Gram-negative bacilli
Coliforms, pseudomonas and serratia are important causes of endocarditis in drug addicts and in patients with prosthetic valves especially during the first few months after cardiac surgery (Tables 2 and 3).

Fungi
Fungal endocarditis is rare but is increasingly recognised as an important problem in patients who have had cardiac surgery and in drug addicts (Tables 2 and 3).

Coxiella burnetti
Q fever endocarditis is rare but must be considered in all cases of blood culture negative endocarditis since its management is radically different from that of bacterial endocarditis.

Chlamydia psittaci
Psittacosis can rarely result in endocarditis and as with Q fever endocarditis the management of patients with this disease is different from that of bacterial endocarditis. The possibility of this disease must always be remembered when the blood cultures are negative.

IMPORTANCE OF ESTABLISHING A MICROBIAL DIAGNOSIS

The mortality of infective endocarditis is greatest in those patients who are given chemotherapy without a microbial diagnosis having been established[1 8 9]. Rational chemotherapy of endocarditis is based on a microbiological diagnosis. Once the infecting organism is known and its susceptibility to relevant chemotherapeutic agents determined, effective treatment can be selected.

A summary of the procedures that are necessary for establishing a microbiological diagnosis is included in Table 6.

Table 6 Microbiological diagnosis of infective endocarditis

Blood culture

(a) 3 routine sets for aerobes and anaerobes, during first 24 h of investigation, before chemotherapy

(b) Further special blood cultures for fastidious organisms when 'blood culture negative endocarditis'

Serology

Paired sera for:
(a) Q fever C.F.T., phase 1 and 2
(b) *Chlamydia psittaci* C.F.T.
(c) Brucella C.F.T.
(d) Fungal precipitins (candida and aspergillus)
(e) Immunofluorescent test for detecting streptococcal antibodies

Other tests

When surgery for removal of infected valve or embolus, microscopy and culture of vegetations or embolus

---

Blood cultures

Blood cultures, 3 sets over a 24 h period, should be collected before the start of antibiotic therapy. Characteristically, the bacteraemia in bacterial endocarditis is constant and low grade. If the patient is acutely ill and needs immediate chemotherapy, 3 sets of cultures can be collected over a 1–2 h period before chemotherapy. Unfortunately some patients have been given antibiotics before investigation. It was recently claimed that the effect of previous antibiotics causing negative blood cultures has been exaggerated[10]. These authors found that positive blood cultures were obtained in 91% of patients with confirmed streptococcal endocarditis who had been given antibiotics within the previous 2 weeks. However, in general it is impossible to know whether antibiotics are responsible for causing negative cultures in *unconfirmed* streptococcal endocarditis cases. When antibiotics have been given they should be stopped and blood cultures, 3 sets in 24 h, repeated every other day for up to 1–2 weeks.

When blood cultures are negative special additional blood culture techniques for isolating fastidious organisms can be selected by the microbiologist when indicated. Special methods that may be necessary include those for the isolation of certain pyridoxine dependent streptococci, haemophilus, lactobacilli, brucella organisms and L forms[11]. Blood culture techniques are reviewed elsewhere[12].

Serology
Serology is essential in all cases of blood culture negative endocarditis and when blood cultures are yielding growth of uncertain clinical significance. An acute specimen of serum should be stored from all patients with suspected endocarditis in case it is needed later, together with a convalescent serum for serology. Serological tests for Q fever, psittacosis and fungi are included in Table 6. An immunofluorescent test for detecting antibodies against viridans streptococci has recently been reported[13].

Duration of investigations
The length of time that can be allowed for investigation of infective endocarditis before starting chemotherapy depends mainly on the severity of the general illness of the patient. Acutely ill cases will need immediate treatment after collection of blood cultures but in many other cases it is desirable to delay treatment for several days until a microbial diagnosis has been made.

GENERAL GUIDELINES FOR EFFECTIVE CHEMOTHERAPY

Bactericidal therapy
Complete bactericidal therapy is essential so that all of the organisms in the endocardial vegetations are killed. The microbiologist can assist greatly in all cases with positive blood cultures by performing appropriate tests on the organism. These include synergy tests when necessary so that the most suitable bactericidal antibiotics can be selected. Also during treatment the laboratory can check that adequate serum bactericidal titres are maintained against the patient's blood culture isolate by a back titration method. Bactericidal titres in the serum against the patient's own organism should be maintained at least at 1/4 for a pre-dose serum and at least at 1/8 for a peak post-dose serum. Further details of laboratory tests and their interpretation are given by Waterworth[14 15].

Duration of treatment
Having determined the choice and dosage of bactericidal antibiotics it is important to continue therapy for long enough to control the infection and reduce the risk of relapse after treatment has stopped. Oakley[6] states that the absolute minimum duration of treatment should be 3 weeks and when a prosthetic valve is present at least 6 weeks. The duration of treatment depends on the infecting organism and also on the rapidity of

clinical response to treatment. In my opinion no patient with infective endocarditis should be treated for less than 4 weeks.

Chemotherapy combined with surgery
Some types of infective endocarditis cannot be adequately treated by chemotherapy alone and surgical excision of an infected valve or foreign material in the heart is also necessary. Examples include Q fever, fungal, and most cases of prosthetic valve endocarditis.

CHOICE OF CHEMOTHERAPEUTIC AGENT DURING BLIND THERAPY
Blind treatment is often necessary while waiting for the results of microbiological investigations and also for those cases where no microbial diagnosis can be made. The choice of agents depends chiefly on the likely microbial aetiology. Suggestions for blind therapy are included in Table 7.

Cases without previous cardiac surgery
Benzyl penicillin given alone has a good therapeutic effect on most cases of streptococcal endocarditis where the infecting organisms are viridans streptococci but it would prove inadequate therapy for endocarditis due to *Streptococcus faecalis,* which is usually less sensitive to penicillin. To cover the latter organism, gentamicin or another aminoglycoside should be added to obtain bactericidal synergy with penicillin.

Staphylococcus aureus strains are usually penicillinase producers[16] and *Staphylococcus aureus* endocarditis does not, therefore, respond to penicillin treatment alone. Gentamicin has useful anti-staphylococcal activity against most penicillinase producing strains although it is not recommended as the drug of choice for staphylococcal infection[17]. If there is clinical evidence to suggest a staphylococcal rather than a streptococcal cause of endocarditis – recent skin sepsis or septicaemia with disseminated intravascular coagulation – large doses of cloxacillin should be used 'blind' together with gentamicin from the beginning of therapy.

Prosthetic valve endocarditis
Gram-positive bacteria constitute the majority of likely infecting organisms at all stages after cardiac surgery. Cloxacillin, penicillin or ampicillin, and gentamicin together should be effective against most staphylococci, diphtheroids and streptococci.

Gram-negative bacilli vary greatly in their antimicrobial sensitivity characteristics. Gentamicin is active against the majority of

Table 7 Blind chemotherapy of bacterial endocarditis

Clinical situation	Main likely organisms	Choice of drug	Dosage and administration	
I. No previous cardiac surgery (but not drug addict)	'Viridans streptococci' Enterococci	Benzyl penicillin plus	16 mega units/day	Intravenous (intermittent 4–6 hourly)
	Staphylococcus aureus†	Gentamicin	80 mg, 8 hourly	Intramuscular
II. Prosthetic valve endocarditis (a) Early onset	Staphylococci	Cloxacillin plus	12 g/day	Intravenous (4 hourly bolus)
	Diphtheroids	Benzyl penicillin plus	12 mega units/day	Intravenous (bolus)
		Gentamicin	80 mg, 6 hourly	Intramuscular
(b) Late onset	Gram-negative bacilli 'Viridans streptococci'	Benzyl penicillin plus	16 mega units/day	Intravenous (intermittent)
		Gentamicin plus	80 mg, 8 hourly	Intramuscular
	Enterococci		8 g/day	Intravenous (4 hourly bolus)
	Staphylococci	Cloxacillin	12 g/day	Intravenous (4 hourly bolus)
III. Drug addict (no previous cardiac surgery)	Staphylococci	Cloxacillin plus	12 g/day	Intravenous
	Gram-negative bacilli	Gentamicin plus	80 mg, 8 hourly	Intramuscular
	Streptococci	Ampicillin	1 g, 4 hourly	Intravenous

† When clinical clues suggest *Staphylococcus aureus* add cloxacillin

enterobacteria and pseudomonas strains and has been useful in the treatment of Gram-negative prosthetic valve endocarditis[18].

Cephalothin, 2 g every 4 h, together with penicillin, 20 mega units intravenously daily and streptomycin, 0.5 g every 12 h intramuscularly is an alternative blind regimen which is used at the New York Hospital, Cornell Medical Center[19]. This regimen is directed at the likely Gram-positive bacteria.

Cephalothin combined with gentamicin provides good cover against both Gram-positive and Gram-negative organisms but this combination is associated with an unacceptable risk of nephrotoxicity[20]. Perhaps one of the newer cephalosporins combined with gentamicin will provide a useful and safe alternative for the blind treatment for prosthetic valve endocarditis in the future. One such possible combination would be cefoxitin combined with gentamicin.

Endocarditis in drug addicts
Immediate blind therapy is mandatory in affected heroin addicts. *Staphylococcus aureus* is the main organism to be covered by therapy with cloxacillin plus gentamicin. When Gram-negative bacilli or mixed infections are present, formidable therapeutic challenges arise and treatment may not be effective until a microbial diagnosis assists rational therapy.

CHOICE OF CHEMOTHERAPEUTIC AGENT ONCE A MICROBIAL DIAGNOSIS HAS BEEN ESTABLISHED IN MEDICAL CASES

Viridans streptococci fully sensitive to penicillin
Benzyl penicillin, given alone, has stood the test of time as the mainstay of treatment of endocarditis due to viridans streptococci which are nearly always fully sensitive to penicillin, (MIC 0.12 mg/l or less)[4 21 22]. The duration of treatment and dosage together determine the effectiveness of penicillin treatment and the relapse rate. Even with the best regimens the mortality rate[1 23] of endocarditis due to these streptococci is 10–15%. The cause of death today is rarely due to lack of control of infection, but is from complications like heart failure, embolic phenomena and renal disease.

The relapse rate in patients treated with large doses of parenteral penicillin alone for 4 weeks has been stated[23–25] to be between 5 and 11%. Some authors suggest that an aminoglycoside should be combined with penicillin to treat endocarditis due to viridans streptococci[5 25–28]. Whether an aminoglycoside should or should not be added to penicillin for treatment is increasingly controversial. Arguments in favour include the greater rapidity of killing streptococci *in vitro*[26] and in experimental rabbit endocarditis[29] [30] when streptomycin is added to penicillin compared with penicillin alone. Clinical evidence of an advantage of adding streptomycin is seen when a course of treatment lasts for only 2 weeks. There are lower relapse rates with the penicillin and streptomycin combination than with penicillin alone following this short period of therapy[28] [31] [32]. Wolfe and Johnson[26] recommended 2 weeks combined penicillin and streptomycin treatment followed by a further 2 weeks parenteral penicillin treatment. These authors state that they have treated over 100 patients with streptococcal endocarditis at the New York Hospital in this way without a single relapse[26]. There is general agreement that ototoxicity occurring during this schedule of treatment with streptomycin is rare.

Oral therapy has been recommended with amoxycillin for fully sensitive viridans streptococci with good results[33]. Oakley[6] has reservations about abandoning parenteral penicillin therapy because of the fear of unacceptably high relapse rates after oral amoxycillin until further work has been done. I feel that oral amoxycillin is useful as a well absorbed penicillin drug to complete a course of treatment between the 2nd and 5th weeks but that at present parenteral benzyl penicillin should be used alone for the first 2 weeks of treatment.

Amoxycillin combined with gentamicin provides optimal bactericidal synergy for most streptococci[22]. A combination that probably would deserve future study would be oral amoxycillin treatment for 5 weeks with injections of gentamicin added during the first 2 weeks of treatment.

Viridans streptococci with reduced sensitivity to penicillin
A few strains of viridans streptococci have a reduced sensitivity to penicillin with an MIC or MBC greater than 0.12 mg per litre. Endocarditis due to these strains should be treated by a combination of penicillin and an aminoglycoside[25].

Streptococcus bovis
Streptococcus bovis causes up to 10% of endocarditis cases[34-36]. This organism is a particularly important cause of endocarditis in patients over the age of 55 years. The great majority of strains are highly sensitive to penicillin although occasional strains have been found with reduced sensitivity to penicillin[37]. The treatment of endocarditis due to *Streptococcus bovis* strains with a MBC to penicillin of less than 0.12 mg/l should be the same as for penicillin sensitive viridans streptococci. Endocarditis due to strains less sensitive to penicillin (MBC greater

than 0.12 mg/l), should be treated by a combination of penicillin and an aminoglycoside as for *Streptococcus faecalis*. There is a possible association between *Streptococcus bovis* endocarditis and carcinoma of the colon[38] [39].

Streptococcus faecalis

In a recent report[2] *Streptococcus faecalis* was the causative organism in 8% of endocarditis cases and was commoner in males. Endocarditis due to *Streptococcus faecalis* is commoner in more elderly patients[40]. The incidence of *Streptococcus faecalis* endocarditis is probably not increasing[7].

A total bactericidal effect against *Streptococcus faecalis* is rarely possible when penicillin or ampicillin or amoxycillin is used alone[22]. A high concentration of penicillin, greater than 6 mg/l, is usually necessary to kill the majority of the population of organisms but survivors occur[41], Aminoglycosides must be added to the penicillin for a complete bactericidal effect and streptomycin has been used for this purpose for many years[42] [43]. The effectiveness of penicillin combined with streptomycin has also been demonstrated in experimental enterococcal endocarditis in dogs[44]. The most usual treatment has consisted of benzyl penicillin, 20 megaunits intravenously daily. for 6 weeks, combined with streptomycin, 1 g intramuscularly every 12 h, for the first 2 or 3 weeks, followed by 0.5 g every 12 h, for the remaining weeks. With penicillin/streptomycin combinations, cure rates of over 80% have been claimed[27] [45] [46].

Bactericidal synergy between penicillin and streptomycin can only be demonstrated when an enterococcus shows some sensitivity to streptomycin[47], apart from some exceptional strains, and recently Basker and Sutherland found that about half the enterococci examined were highly resistant to streptomycin[22]. These authors invariably found that enterococci were partially sensitive to gentamicin and that bactericidal synergy between penicillin and gentamicin could always be demonstrated. Possible antibiotic combinations that may need to be considered for the treatment of a difficult *Streptococcus faecalis* endocarditis are included in Table 8.

Ampicillin or amoxycillin have slightly greater activity than penicillin against most *Streptococcus faecalis* strains and the most potent bactericidal combination *in vitro* against enterococci appears to be amoxycillin plus gentamicin[22]. Amoxycillin can now be given by injection and for at least the first 2 weeks of treatment this is advisable. There are no clinical data so far to show that the theoretical advantages of gentamicin compared with streptomycin are born out in practice.

Table 8 Possible antibiotic combinations for achieving complete bactericidal therapy for *Streptococcus faecalis* endocarditis

Penicillin drug or Vancomycin	plus	Aminoglycoside
Benzyl penicillin or Ampicillin or Amoxycillin or Vancomycin		Streptomycin or Gentamicin or Kanamycin or Tobramycin or Amikacin or Sisomicin or Netilmicin

The risk of toxic effects from an aminoglycoside should be minimised by frequent monitoring of the serum levels during treatment so that the dosage can be modified if necessary. If gentamicin is used serum trough levels should not exceed 2 mg/l.

I think that benzyl penicillin or amoxycillin should be given parenterally combined with gentamicin for the treatment of *Streptococcus faecalis* endocarditis until further information on the antimicrobial sensitivities of the isolate is available. If renal function is impaired streptomycin may be substituted for gentamicin provided that the *Streptococcus faecalis* is partially sensitive to streptomycin and that synergy with penicillin can be demonstrated. The level of streptomycin should be assayed frequently in order to avoid toxic effects on the eighth cranial nerve. For those *Streptococcus faecalis* isolates where there is a high level of resistance to streptomycin and synergy can be shown with a penicillin plus gentamicin combination, the gentamicin combination should be continued even when there is impairment of renal function.

Staphylococcus aureus

Staphylococcus aureus usually causes an acute endocarditis that is rapidly fatal unless appropriate, prompt bactericidal treatment is given. Benzyl penicillin is the drug of choice when isolates are fully sensitive to penicillin. However, penicillinase-producing strains of *Staphylococcus aureus* are more common and these are nearly always sensitive to cloxacillin and gentamicin. High doses of cloxacillin are necessary, 2 g intravenously every 4 h. Cloxacillin alone may not be completely bactericidal[21] and gentamicin should be added at the same time, in a dosage of 80 mg, 8 hourly, intramuscularly. Gentamicin is nearly always the best aminoglycoside to add to obtain bactericidal synergy but extensive synergy testing should be performed on each isolate to find the best antibiotic combination. The range of antibiotics used in combination testing should include, penicillins, methicillin group, cephalosporins, aminoglycosides, rifampicin, fucidin, erythromycin and vancomycin. It is essential to ensure that bactericidal serum levels are maintained during treatment to a dilution of at least 1 in 8. Experimental work has shown that gentamicin added to nafcillin, a β-lactam drug resistant to penicillinase, accelerated the eradication of staphylococci from cardiac vegetations in rabbits[48]. When methicillin resistant strains of *Staphylococcus aureus* cause endocarditis, vancomycin may be useful in therapy[49].

Fucidin added to cloxacillin has been recommended for the treatment of *Staphylococcus aureus* endocarditis when the organism is sensitive to both these drugs[6]. *In vitro* data with some strains of *Staphylococcus aureus* shows that antagonism can occur when fucidin is combined with penicillin drugs[50] and some bacteriologists prefer not to use this combination in the treatment of *Staphylococcus aureus* endocarditis.

Haemophilus

Although streptococci and staphylococci cause over 80% of infective endocarditis the importance of haemophilus as a cause of endocarditis has become increasingly recognised in younger adult patients due to improved blood culture techniques[51]. *Haemophilus parainfluenzae* and *aphrophilus* are the species most frequently isolated from blood cultures[52] [53]. *Haemophilus influenzae* and *paraphrophilus* are less frequent causes of endocarditis.

Ampicillin plus gentamicin for 6–8 weeks is the treatment usually recommended for haemophilus endocarditis but good results have been claimed for ampicillin alone, 12 g daily for 3 weeks, when the strains isolated are fully sensitive to ampicillin[54]. However, a recent case report suggested that ampicillin alone may not be adequate for *Haemophilus parainfluenzae* sensitive to ampicillin[55].

Anaerobes

Recently bacteroides, fusobacterium and anaerobic cocci have been isolated more frequently from endocarditis cases. This is probably because of improved anaerobic blood culture techniques. An American review[56] showed that anaerobes can cause a particularly invasive and destructive type of endocarditis. Fusobacteria and anaerobic cocci are usually sensitive to benzyl penicillin or ampicillin which should be given in large doses intravenously. *Bacteroides fragilis* produces a β-lactamase so penicillin drugs should not be used for treating endocarditis due to this species.

Metronidazole has great bactericidal activity against all the non-sporing anaerobic bacteria[57] [58]. This valuable drug can be used to treat all cases of anaerobic endocarditis either alone or in combination with other bactericidal antibiotics. Fusobacterium endocarditis has been successfully treated with a combination of ampicillin and metronidazole[59].

Cardiobacterium hominis

Cardiobacterium hominis is an infrequent but well recognised cause of endocarditis. A recent report suggests that 3 weeks of therapy with benzyl penicillin or ampicillin alone is adequate therapy[60].

Lactobacilli

Lactobacillus casei endocarditis is rarely reported. This may be due partly to the exacting blood culture methods necessary for the isolation of lactobacilli. Treatment with penicillin and streptomycin, given together in large doses, has proved successful in several cases[61].

Coxiella burnetti

Q fever endocarditis is very rare and although Q fever is a world wide disease it is remarkable that most of the cases have been reported from Britain[62].

Tetracycline treatment alone may improve the general condition of the patient but the coxiella organism will not be eradicated from cardiac vegetations by tetracycline; surgical intervention to replace the infected valve is almost always necessary in addition to tetracycline treatment[63]. After surgery, continued tetracycline treatment should be given for at least 2 years. Prolonged surveillance is necessary because the prosthetic valve may become infected by the same organism a long time after surgery[64 65].

Co-trimoxazole has also been used to treat Q fever endocarditis but experience with this drug is limited[66].

Chlamydia psittaci

The psittacosis agent was first reported to have caused infective endocarditis in 1971[67]. Treatment with tetracycline is indicated and surgical removal of the infected valve has proved necessary in one case[68]. The management of this rare condition should probably be similar to that outlined above for Q fever endocarditis.

CHOICE OF CHEMOTHERAPY WHEN A MICROBIAL DIAGNOSIS IS ESTABLISHED IN CASES OF PROSTHETIC VALVE ENDOCARDITIS

The chemotherapy of prosthetic valve endocarditis is the same as for endocarditis in medical cases, with one major exception. This exception is '*Streptococcus viridans*' endocarditis, which is the most common cause of late onset infection of the prosthetic heart valve. I suggest that a combination of penicillin and an aminoglycoside be given in this situation even when the viridans streptococci are fully sensitive to penicillin. More rapid control of the infection might be expected on the theoretical grounds already discussed by using penicillin alone. In some cases the combination chemotherapy of *Streptococcus viridans* prosthetic valve endocarditis has been so successful that surgery has proved unnecessary[69]. In most cases, however, surgical removal of the infected valve is essential to obtain a permanent cure.

Staphylococcus epidermidis (albus)

About a third of all cases of prosthetic valve endocarditis are caused by *Staphylococcus epidermidis*[19] which may present either as early or late onset endocarditis. When *Staphylococcus epidermidis* strains are sensitive to it, methicillin 2 g intravenously every 4 h for 4–6 weeks has been recommended[69]. Cephalothin, 2 g intravenously every 4 h, is an alternative if necessary. When strains are sensitive to methicillin and gentamicin this combination is preferred using a regimen as for *Staphylococcus aureus* endocarditis.

Many strains of coagulase negative staphylococci are resistant to methicillin but American workers claim that these may be sensitive to cephalosporins[70]. Some microbiologists claim that there is cross resistance between methicillin resistant staphylococci and cephalosporins and more work is necessary on this subject. Cephradine is highly active against β-lactamase producing strains of staphylococci[71], but its value in the treatment of *Staphylococcus epidermidis* endocarditis has yet to be determined. Vancomycin may be valuable in the treatment of methicillin resistant *Staphylococcus epidermidis* endocarditis[19].

Suppression of the infection can be continued with antibiotics for many months but a relapse may occur when the treatment is stopped, unless the infected valve is removed[72 73].

Diphtheroid bacilli

Aerobic and anaerobic diphtheroids are important causes of endocarditis, particularly during the first 2 months after heart surgery although they cause prosthetic valve endocarditis much less frequently than staphylococci or Gram-negative bacilli. Combination antibiotic therapy consisting of penicillin or erythromycin plus streptomycin or gentamicin, has been recommended until the antibiotic sensitivities of the diphtheroid strain are ascertained[74]. When the strain isolated is very sensitive to penicillin, treatment can be given with penicillin alone, although some cardiologists prefer to give an aminoglycoside also in this situation.

About one third of diphtheroids are resistant to both penicillin and cephalosporins. These strains are often sensitive to vancomycin which has been used successfully in treatment[19 75].

Gram-negative bacilli

Gram-negative bacilli were responsible for 33% of prosthetic valve endocarditis cases in one series[69] and in this series 83% of patients who had early onset Gram-negative endocarditis died. Most of the cases of Gram-negative endocarditis occur within 2 months of surgery, but late onset Gram-negative endocarditis also occurs[19]. The most frequent organisms implicated are *Klebsiella, Escherichia, Pseudomonas, Serratia* and *Proteus* spp. Effective treatment of Gram-negative endocarditis is notoriously difficult. Combinations of antibiotics are usually necessary, preferably bactericidal antibiotics, and the choice depends on the results of antibiotic sensitivity tests[49]. Trimethoprim plus sulphonamides[76] and ampicillin plus kanamycin[77] have been effective. I suggest a combination of ampicillin plus gentamicin when the causative organism is sensitive to both these antibiotics. Multiple antibiotic resistant strains of Gram-negative bacilli, including gentamicin resistant negative bacilli, are often sensitive to the newer cephalosporins, cefuroxime and cefoxitin. These last two cephalosporins may have a useful place in the future treatment of Gram-negative endocarditis used alone or in combination with aminoglycosides.

Salmonellae may cause prosthetic valve endocarditis of late onset – sometimes years after successful valve replacement. Mecillinam in combination with a β-lactam antibiotic may be useful for treating salmonella endocarditis[78]. The mortality of salmonella endocarditis is high and early removal of the infected valve is usually necessary.

Pseudomonas cepacia prosthetic valve endocarditis has been treated with a combination of rifampicin, co-trimoxazole and cephalexin[79].

Fungi
Fungal endocarditis following open heart surgery has been increasingly recognised during the last 15 years[80-84].

Most of the early reports of treatment of candida endocarditis describe the use of intravenous amphotericin B alone and are associated with a high mortality rate[85]. This drug is fungistatic rather than fungicidal and may cause serious nephrotoxicity but good results have been obtained in conjunction with urgent surgical removal of the infected valve[86]. An alternative drug to amphotericin B is 5-fluorocytosine which is also fungistatic rather than fungicidal and some success has been reported using this drug[87]. 5-fluorocytosine is less toxic than amphotericin B although harmful side effects on the liver and bone marrow may be produced. A combination of amphotericin B and 5-fluorocytosine has been suggested for the treatment of candida endocarditis[88]. When this combination is used the development of resistance of the yeasts to 5-fluorocytosine during treatment is less likely. A further advantage of giving the combination is that the dose of amphotericin B can be reduced so that the chances of side effects occurring are reduced. 5-fluorocytosine has no activity against filamentous fungi and the treatment of aspergillus endocarditis can only be seriously attempted at the present time through a combination of intravenous amphotericin B and surgery.

Follow-up of treated cases of prosthetic valve endocarditis
Chemotherapy may need to be continued for many months in some cases of prosthetic valve endocarditis even when an infected valve has been excised. When patients are well, treatment can be given at home but frequent outpatient visits are essential. Once treatment has been stopped, a monthly follow-up as an outpatient is usually advisable. Blood cultures may also be collected, for up to 1 year.

HYPERSENSITIVITY TO PENICILLIN

Penicillin is the drug of choice for treating many cases of bacterial endocarditis. When a patient develops allergy to penicillin it is best to continue penicillin treatment under antihistamine and steroid cover whenever possible[89]. Steroid therapy does not altogether remove the chance of anaphylaxis but the risk of this happening can probably be reduced by increasing the penicillin dose gradually[90].

Cephalosporins have frequently been used to treat endocarditis due to viridans streptococci when patients develop penicillin allergy. However it should also be remembered that a few penicillin hypersensitive patients may also be hypersensitive to cephalosporins[91]. Cephaloridine, cephalothin, and cephazolin have been successfully used to treat endocarditis due to viridans streptococci[92].

Endocarditis due to *Streptococcus faecalis* should not be treated by cephalosporins because *in vitro* and in experimental endocarditis in rabbits, cephalosporins have an inadequate bactericidal effect against the organism, even when in combination with aminoglycosides[93][94]. It is, therefore, particularly important to continue penicillin treatment, in conjunction with aminoglycosides, even when there is penicillin allergy by taking suitable precautions. Desensitization to penicillin has been suggested[95] and if this fails steroid cover may suppress reactions. If severe toxic effects develop in spite of these various measures the penicillin must be stopped and vancomycin may be used instead[96][97].

Patients with staphylococcal endocarditis may receive treatment with cephalosporins instead of the cloxacillin group of drugs when there is penicillin allergy. Cephalosporins have proved to be effective in the treatment of *Staphylococcus aureus* endocarditis either alone or in combination with other antibiotics[98-100]. Cephradine is particularly resistant to staphylococcal β-lactamase[71] and has been successfully used to treat *Staphylococcus aureus* endocarditis[101].

ADMINISTRATION OF DRUGS

Intravenous therapy is nearly always necessary at the start of treatment. Thorough aseptic and antiseptic techniques are important as infection at the drip site, often staphylococcal or fungal, must be avoided. Thin walled butterfly needles in peripheral veins, changed at 48 h intervals, are recommended.

I prefer bolus administration rather than the continuous intravenous infusion of antibiotics to patients with endocarditis but there are no clear data at present that this is preferable.

The oral administration of antibiotics, with or without probenecid, has been discussed previously but it is worth stressing that frequent determinations of the serum bactericidal titre against the patient's own organisms are necessary to ensure that adequate doses are given.

PERSISTENT PYREXIA DURING THE TREATMENT

A persistent pyrexia during antibiotic treatment should lead one to suspect either (a) development of a drug reaction; (b) super-infection; (c) infection of the intravenous line; (d) lack of control of the original infection by chemotherapy; (e) a combination of one or more of the above. Further blood cultures are indicated followed by replacement of the intravenous line and culture of the tip. Should the pyrexia continue and the cause remain unclear, the drugs should be stopped. When the pyrexia is due to a drug reaction the temperature rapidly returns to normal and the drugs may be restarted taking the appropriate precautions discussed previously.

INDICATIONS FOR SURGERY

In the last 13 years the value of surgery in the management of endocarditis has become increasingly recognised. Various haemodynamic complications, such as severe aortic regurgitation, may indicate the need for surgery. When these complications occur suddenly, emergency surgery is often necessary. Ideally, surgery should be performed when the patient is not in heart failure and when there is no longer any infection at the site of the heart valve. These ideal conditions may exist in those patients who have only slowly developed haemodynamic complications.

Some infections are not controlled by chemotherapy alone. These include most infections of prosthetic heart valves particularly when the causative organisms are Gram-negative bacilli, staphylococci, and fungi. Q fever and psittacosis endocarditis are not cured by the bacteristatic agent tetracycline alone and surgical excision of the infected valve is essential.

This important subject is extensively reviewed elsewhere[3] [102] [103].

CHEMOPROPHYLAXIS OF ENDOCARDITIS

Most types of rheumatic, congenital and atherosclerotic heart disease may predispose to infective endocarditis and these are discussed fully in a recent statement from the American Heart Association concerning prophylaxis[104]. An important aspect of prophylaxis concerns the prevention of bacteraemia by methods not using antibiotics. These methods include a high standard of oral hygiene to reduce the chances of dental bacteraemia from diseased gums or teeth. Also in patients with prosthetic valves good food hygiene is important to prevent salmonella endocarditis. The most important indication for chemoprophylaxis is to prevent endocarditis following the bacteraemia associated with dental extractions.

Dental procedures
The risk of bacterial endocarditis developing in a susceptible patient after dental extraction has been estimated[105] at about 1 in 500. There are no scientifically controlled data to show that prophylaxis is effective in the prevention of 'dental' endocarditis in man because endocarditis is too uncommon for worthwhile trials to be undertaken. Circumstantial evidence demands that chemoprophylaxis should be given; the oral organisms that enter the blood after extraction are the same as those that may cause endocarditis in susceptible subjects and endocarditis is associated with serious morbidity and mortality. Chemoprophylaxis is indicated for dental extractions and also any other procedures that are expected to cause gingival bleeding[104].

The choice of antibiotics for prophylaxis should take some account of the recent data from experimental endocarditis in rabbits[106] [107]. These experiments showed that bacteristatic agents such as tetracycline and many other antibiotics including co-trimoxazole and cephalexin are unsuitable. For effective chemoprophylaxis it appears essential to have both high serum bactericidal levels of antibiotic at the expected time of bacteraemia and also persistent serum bactericidal levels for the duration of a critical period which lasts from 6–9 h following bacteraemia. There is little evidence that prophylaxis should exceed 24 h though it is traditional to suggest a 48 h period of prophylaxis following bacteraemia. It is important not to start the chemoprophylaxis too soon before extraction as antibiotic resistant strains of bacteria may be selected[108].

Parenteral antibiotics are generally preferable to oral drugs[109 110], but in practice oral antibiotics often are given[111 112].

My recommendations for the prophylaxis of endocarditis in dental patients are given in Table 9. Some of the recommendations of the American Heart Association possibly adhere too closely to the rabbit experimental endocarditis data and I do not accept that streptomycin is necessary in addition to penicillin for every susceptible patient when the gums are expected to bleed. However, there are many valuable aspects in the American recommendations, particularly the need to give a sufficiently large loading dose of penicillin V, 2 g, when oral prophylaxis needs to be given. I recommend amoxycillin, 2 g, instead of penicillin V, 2 g, one hour before extraction because higher and more persistent bactericidal levels are obtained with amoxycillin[113]. In the latter study both penicillin V and amoxycillin, 2 g dosage, were effective in greatly reducing the incidence of bacteraemia following extraction. Some recent work has shown that even larger initial doses of amoxycillin, given as a syrup, may be well tolerated. 3 and 4 g doses of amoxycillin were given to 12 volunteers and produced serum bactericidal levels that persisted for at least 12 h after the dose[114]. In future it appears likely that a single supervised 3–4 g oral dose of amoxycillin given one hour before dental extraction will provide all the effective oral chemoprophylaxis required in susceptible subjects without the need for any further doses after extraction.

Endocarditis in patients with prosthetic heart valves is particularly catastrophic since excision of the valve is frequently necessary. Therefore, I think that a 'belt and braces' approach is desirable with these patients. A further recommendation of the AHA of using streptomycin as well as penicillin by the parenteral route should be adhered to as suggested in Table 9.

Manipulations or surgery on the genito-urinary tract or bowel
Streptococcus faecalis endocarditis may follow instrumentation or surgery on the genito-urinary tract or bowel unless chemoprophylaxis is given. Ampicillin, 1 g intramuscularly or intravenously should be given 15–30 minutes before the procedure plus gentamicin, 80 mg by a separate injection. Repeated injections of each drug can be given 6 and 12 h after the procedure.

For patients allergic to penicillin, erythromycin lactobionate, 300 mg can be given intravenously 15 minutes before the procedure instead of ampicillin and again at 6 and 12 h after the procedure. When the patient

Table 9 Prophylaxis of endocarditis in patients undergoing dental extractions

Medical cases

1st choice– Parenteral prophylaxis
Fortified benzathine penicillin, BPC, I.M. injection, 15–30 minutes before extraction. (Trade name 'Penidural All Purpose' – consists of a mixture of:- penicillin G 190 mg, procaine penicillin G 300 mg, benzathine penicillin 450 mg)

2nd choice – Oral prophylaxis
Amoxycillin capsules or syrup, 2 g, give one hour before extraction, followed by 500 mg, 6 hourly for 24 hours

1st choice when patient allergic to penicillin
Cephazolin 1 g, I.M. injection plus streptomycin 1 g, separate I.M. injection 15–30 minutes before extraction

2nd choice when patient allergic to penicillin
Erythromycin 1 g orally, 30 minutes before extraction, followed by 500 mg 6 hourly for 24 hours

In surgical cases – prosthetic valve present

Parenteral prophylaxis always

1st choice when no penicillin allergy
Fortified benzathine penicillin mixture, I.M. injection, 15–30 minutes before extraction (as for medical cases)

plus

Streptomycin 1 g, as a separate I.M. injection 15–30 minutes before extraction

2nd choice when patient allergic to penicillin
Vancomycin 1 g, intravenously by slow infusion, about 15 minutes before procedure

plus

Streptomycin 1 g, I.M. injection 30 minutes before extraction

is allergic to penicillin and has a prosthetic heart valve, intravenous vancomycin, 1 g, plus gentamicin, 80 mg intramuscularly may be given 20 minutes before the procedure and at 8 and 16 h after the procedure.

Open heart surgery
The organisms most likely to infect the prosthetic heart valve at the time of operation or during the immediate postoperative period include *Staphylococcus aureus, Staphylococcus epidermidis* and diphtheroids, although Gram-negative bacilli may also cause infection as discussed in a previous section. Fungi are rare causes of endocarditis compared to

bacteria and it is not necessary to consider chemoprophylaxis against fungi.

Cloxacillin is active against over 90% of *Staphylococcus aureus* strains and since this agent has been used extensively to provide antibiotic cover at the time of operation and during the immediate postoperative period, *Staphylococcus aureus* endocarditis has become infequent. Many *Staphylococcus epidermidis* strains are resistant to methicillin but sensitive to gentamicin and for this reason, antibiotic prophylaxis for open heart surgery should consist of a combination of cloxacillin and gentamicin. An additional reason for using gentamicin is the cover provided against Gram-negative bacilli.

Diphtheroids may be much more sensitive to penicillin than to either methicillin or aminoglycosides[115]. In order to provide prophylaxis against staphylococci, diphtheroids and Gram-negative bacilli a combination of cloxacillin, benzyl penicillin and gentamicin has been used at Papworth Hospital, England, where no cases of endocarditis have been noted following 800 open heart operations[116]. The first doses of this cocktail are given parenterally with the premedication and by intravenous infusion for up to 48 h after the operation. Newsom has given an excellent overall review of prophylaxis for open heart surgery in this article[116].

The incidence of different antibiotic resistant strains of bacteria is bound to vary between different hospitals and different countries. A rational prophylactic regimen therefore depends to some extent on the local circumstances and full discussions are necessary between the clinician and the microbiologist.

References

1 Hayward, G. W. (1973). Infective endocarditis: a changing disease. *Brit. Med. J.*, **2**, 706

2 Schnurr, L. P., Ball, A. P., Geddes, A. M., Gray, J. and M̈cGhie, D. (1977). Bacterial endocarditis in England in the 1970's. A review of 70 patients. *Q. J. Med.*, **184**, 499

3 Hamer, J. and O'Grady, F. W. (1977). Infective endocarditis. In J. Hamer (ed.) *Recent Advances in Cardiology*. 7th ed. (London: Churchill Livingstone)

4 Cates, J. E. and Christie, R. V. (1951). Subacute bacterial endocarditis. *Q. J. Med.*, **26**, 93

5 Ball, A. P. and Geddes, A. M. (1978). Streptococcal endocarditis: a penicillin alone or a penicillin with an aminoglycoside. *J. Antimicrob. Chemother.*, **4**, 381

6 Oakley, C. (1978). Use of antibiotics: Endocarditis. *Brit. Med. J.*, **2**, 489

7 Parker, M. T. and Ball, L. C. (1976). Streptococci and aerococci associated with systemic infection in man. *J. Med. Microbiol.*, **9**, 277

8 Hampton, J. R. and Harrison, M. J. G. (1967). Sterile blood cultures in bacterial endocarditis. *Q. J. Med.*, **36**, 167

9 Friedberg, C. K. (1964). Endocarditis. *Bull. N.Y. Acad. Med.,* **40,** 522
10 Werner, A. S., Cobbs, C. G., Kaye, D. *et al.* (1967). Studies on the bacteraemia of bacterial endocarditis. *J. Am. Med. Sci.,* **202,** 199
11 Leading Article. (1977). Blood culture negative endocarditis. *Lancet,* **2,** 1164
12 Shanson, D. C. (1978). Blood culture techniques. In J. D. Williams (ed.) *Modern Topics in Infection.* (London: Heinemann)
13 Shanson, D. C. and Hince, C. (1978). An immunofluorescent method for detecting antibodies against viridans streptococci in *Streptococcus viridans* endocarditis. *J. Clin. Pathol.,* **31,** 292
14 Waterworth, P. M. (1973). Laboratory control of antibiotic therapy. In L. P. Garrod, H. P. Lambert and F. O'Grady (eds.) *Antibiotic and Chemotherapy.* (Edinburgh and London: Churchill Livingstone)
15 Waterworth, P. M. (1978). Tests of combined antibacterial action. In D. S. Reeves, I. Phillips, J. D. Williams and R. Wise (eds.) *Laboratory Methods in Antimicrobial Chemotherapy.* (London: Churchill Livingstone)
16 Wise, R. (1978). Use of antibiotics. Penicillins. *Brit. Med. J.,* **1,** 1679
17 Bindt, A. J. (1976). Leading Article. Gentamicin-resistant *Staphylococcus aureus. Antibiot. Microbiol. Chemother.,* **2,** 225
18 Snow, R. M. and Cobbs, C. G. (1974). Infective endocarditis. In H. F. Conn (ed.) *Current Therapy,* pp. 194–201. (Philadelphia: Saunders)
19 Johnson, W. D. (1976). Prosthetic valve endocarditis. In D. Kaye (ed.) *Infective Endocarditis.* (Baltimore: University Park Press)
20 Marsh, F. P. (1978). Do cephalosporins potentiate or antagonize aminoglycoside nephrotoxicity? *J. Antimicrob. Chemother.,* **4,** 577
21 Garrod, L. P., Lambert, H. P. and F. O'Grady (1973). Septicaemia and Endocarditis. *Antibiotic and Chemotherapy* (London: Churchill Livingstone)
22 Basker, M. J. and Sutherland, R. (1977). Activity of amoxycillin, alone, and in combination with aminoglycoside antibiotics against streptococci associated with bacterial endocarditis. *J. Antimicrob. Chemother.,* **3,** 273
23 Hook, E. W. and Guerrant, R. L. (1976). Therapy of infective endocarditis. In D. Kaye (ed.) *Infective Endocarditis.* (Baltimore: University Park Press)
24 Lerner, P. I. and Weinstein, L. (1966). Infective endocarditis in the antibiotic era. *New Engl. J. Med.,* **274,** 199, 259–265, 323, 388
25 Eckhardt, R., Lüthy, R. and Siegenthaler, W. (1978). Penicillin or penicillin/streptomycin therapy in subacute streptococcal endocarditis. In *Current Chemotherapy,* Proceedings of the 10th International Congress of Chemotherapy, September 1977, **1,** 268–269
26 Wolfe, J. C. and Johnson, W. D. (1974). Penicillin sensitive streptococcal endocarditis. *In vitro* and clinical observations on penicillin-streptomycin therapy. *Ann. Intern. Med.,* **81,** 178
27 Kaye, D. (1973). Changes in the spectrum, diagnosis and management of bacterial and fungal endocarditis. *Med. Clin. North. Am.,* **57,** 941
28 Tan, T. S., Terhune, C. A., Kaplan, S. and Hamburger, M. (1971). Successful two week treatment schedule for penicillin susceptible *Streptococcus viridans* endocarditis. *Lancet,* **2,** 1340
29 Durack, D. T. and Petersdorf, R. G. (1973). Chemotherapy of experimental streptococcal endocarditis. Comparison of commonly recommended prophylaxis regimes. *J. Clin. Invest.,* **52,** 592
30 Sande, M. A. and Irwin, R. C. (1974). Penicillin aminoglycoside synergy in experimental *Streptococcus viridans* endocarditis. *J. Infect. Dis.,* **129,** 572
31 Hunter, T. H. and Paterson, P. Y. (1956). Bacterial endocarditis. *Dev. Med.,* **1,** 1

32 Tompsett, R., Robbins, W. C. and Bernsten, C. (1958). Short term penicillin and dihydrostreptomycin therapy of streptococcal endocarditis. *Am. J. Med.,* **24,** 57
33 Gray, I. R. (1975). The choice of antibiotic for treating infective endocarditis. *Q. J. Med.,* **44,** 419
34 Niven, C. F. and White, J. C. (1946). A study of streptococci associated with subacute bacterial endocarditis. *J. Bacteriol.,* **151,** 790
35 Foley, G. E. (1947). Further observations on the occurrence of streptococci of groups other than A in human infection. *New Engl. J. Med.,* **237,** 909
36 Porterfield, J. S. (1950). Classification of the streptococci of subacute bacterial endocarditis. *J. Gen. Microbiol.,* **4,** 92
37 Thornsberry, C., Baker, C. N. and Facklam, R. R. (1974). Antibiotic susceptibility of *Streptococcus bovis* and other group D streptococci causing endocarditis. *Antimicrob. Agents Chemother.,* **5,** 228
38 Klein, R. J., Recco, R. A., Catalano, M. T. *et al.* (1977). Association of *Streptococcus bovis* with carcinoma of the colon. *New Engl. J. Med.,* **297,** 800
39 Noble, C. J., Uttley, A. H., Falk, R. H. and Richardson, P. J. (1978). *Streptococcus bovis* endocarditis and colonic cancer. *Lancet,* **1,** 766
40 Cherubin, C. E. and Neu, H. C. (1971). Infective endocarditis at the Presbyterian Hospital in New York City from 1938–1967. *Am. J. Med.,* **51,** 83
41 Jawetz, E. (1952). Antibiotic synergism and antagonism. Review of experimental evidence. *Arch. Intern. Med.,* **90,** 301
42 Robbins, W. C. and Tompsett, R. (1951). Treatment of enterococcal endocarditis and bacteraemia. Results of combined therapy with penicillin and streptomycin. *Am. J. Med.,* **10,** 279
43 Cates, J. E., Christie, R. V. and Garrod, L. P. (1951). Penicillin resistant subacute bacterial endocarditis treated by a combination of penicillin and streptomycin. *Brit. Med. J.,* **1,** 653
44 Sapico, F. L., Kegs, T. F. and Hewitt, W. L. (1972). Experimental enterococcal endocarditis. II. Study of *in vivo* synergism of penicillin and streptomycin. *Am. J. Med. Sci.,* **263,** 128
45 Mandell, G. L., Kaye, D., Levison, M. E. and Hook, E. W. (1970). Enterococcal endocarditis: an analysis of 38 patients observed at the New York Hospital – Cornell Medical Center. *Arch. Intern. Med.,* **125,** 258
46 Geraci, J. E. and Martin, W. J. (1953). Antibiotic therapy of bacterial endocarditis. *Circulation,* **10,** 173
47 Watanakunakorn, C. (1971). Penicillin combined with gentamicin or streptomycin; synergism against enterococci. *J. Infect. Dis.,* **124,** 581
48 Sande, M. A. and Courtney, K. (1974). Nafcillin-gentamicin synergism in experimental staphylococcal endocarditis. *14th Inter-science Conference on Antimicrobial Agents and Chemotherapy* (Abstract 76)
49 Cannon, N. J. and Cobbs, C. G. (1976). Infective endocarditis in drug addicts. In D. Kaye (ed.) *Infective Endocarditis,* p. 124. (Baltimore: University Park Press)
50 Greenwood, D. and O'Grady, F. (1973). Interactions between fusidic acid and penicillins. *J. Med. Microbiol.,* **6,** 441
51 Leading Article (1977). Haemophilus endocarditis. *Lancet,* **1,** 1349
52 Lynn, D. J., Kane, J. G., Parker, R. H. (1977). *Haemophilus parainfluenzae* and *influenzae* endocarditis: a review of forty cases. *Medicine,* **56,** 115
53 Johnson, R. H., Kennedy, R. P., Morton, K. I. and Thornsberry, C. (1977). *Haemophilus endocarditis:* new cases, literature review and recommendations for management. *South Med. J.,* **70,** 1098
54 Geraci, J. E., Wilkowske, C. J., Wilson, W. R. and Washington, J. A. (1977).

Haemophilus endocarditis. Report of 14 patients. *Mayo Clinic Proc.*, **52**, 209

55 Ree, G. H., Mundodi, B., and Martin, C. M. (1977). Haemophilus endocarditis. *Lancet*, **2**, 305

56 Nastro, L. J. and Finegold, J. M. (1973). Endocarditis due to anaerobic Gram-negative bacilli. *Am. J. Med.*, **54**, 482

57 Chow, A. W., Patten, V. and Guze, L. B. (1975). Susceptibility of anaerobic bacteria to metronidazole: relative resistance of non-spore-forming Gram-positive bacilli. *J. Infect. Dis.*, **131**, 182

58 Tally, F. P., Sutter, V. L. and Finegold, S. M. (1975). Treatment of anaerobic infections with metronidazole. *Antimicrob. Agents Chemother.*, **7**, 672

59 Seggie, J. (1978). Fusobacterium endocarditis treated with metronidazole. *Brit. Med. J.*, **1**, 960

60 Geraci, J. E., Greipp, P. R., Wilkowske, C. J., Wilson, W. R. and Washington, J. A. II. (1978). *Cardiobacterium hominis* endocarditis. Four cases with clinical and laboratory observations. *Mayo Clinic Proc.*, **53**, 49

61 Isenberg, D. (1977). Lactobacillus infective endocarditis. *Proc. R. Soc. Med.*, **70**, 278

62 Leading Article. (1976). Q fever endocarditis. *Brit. Med. J.*, **2**, 960

63 Kristinsson, A. and Bentall, H. H. (1967). Medical and surgical treatment of Q fever endocarditis. *Lancet*, **2**, 693

64 Turck, W. P., Howitt, G., Turnberg, L. A. *et al.* (1976). Chronic Q fever. *Q. J. Med.*, **45**, 193

65 Tunstall Pedoe, H. D. (1970). Apparent recurrence of Q fever endocarditis following homograft replacement of aortic valve. *Brit. Heart J.*, **32**, 568

66 Freeman, R. and Hodson, M. E. (1972). Q fever endocarditis treated with trimethoprim and sulphamethoxazole. *Brit. Med. J.*, **1**, 419

67 Levison, D. A., Ward, C., Guthrie, W. W., Green, D. M., and Robertson, P. G. C. (1971). Infective endocarditis as part of Psittacosis. *Lancet*, **2**, 844

68 Birkhead, J. S. and Apostolov, K. (1974). Endocarditis caused by a psittacosis agent. *Brit. Heart J.*, **36**, 728

69 Wilson, W. E., Jaumin, P. M., Danielson, G. K., Giuliani, E. R., Washington, J. A. and Geraci, J. E. (1975). Prosthetic valve endocarditis. *Ann. Intern. Med.*, **82**, 751

70 Weinstein, L. and Rubin, R. H. (1973). Infective endocarditis. *Prog. Cardiovasc. Dis.*, **16**, 239

71 Selwyn, S. (1977). Susceptibility of penicillins and cephalosporins to Beta-lactamases assessed by a new test. *J. Antimicrob. Chemother.*, **3**, 161

72 Watanakunakorn, C. and Hamburger, M. (1970). Staphylococcus epidermidis endocarditis complicating a Starr Edwards Prosthesis. *Arch. Int. Med.*, **126**, 1014

73 Fraser, R. S., Rossall, R. E., and Dvorkin, J. (1967). Bacterial endocarditis occurring after open heart surgery. *Canad. Med. Assoc. J.*, **96**, 1551

74 Gerry, J. L. and Greenough III, W. B. (1976). Diphtheroid endocarditis. Report of 9 cases and review of the literature. *The Johns Hopkins Medical Journal*, **139**, 61

75 Johnson, W. D. and Kaye, D. (1970). Serious infections caused by diptheroids. *Ann. N.Y. Acad. Sci.*, **174**, 568

76 Fowle, A. S. E. and Zorab, C. A. (1970). *E. coli* endocarditis successfully treated with oral trimethoprim and sulphamethoxazole. *Brit. Heart J.*, **32**, 127

77 Hansing, C. E., Allen, V. D. and Cherry, J. D. (1967). *E. coli* endocarditis. A review of the literature and a case study. *Arch. Int. Med.*, **120**, 472

78 Shanson, D. C., Brigden, W. and Weaver, E. J. M. (1977). *Salmonella enteritidis* endocarditis. *Brit. Med. J.*, **1**, 612

79 Phillips, I. and Eykyn, S. (1973). Bacterial endocarditis following heart surgery. In

A. M. Geddes and J. D. Williams (eds.) *Current Antibiotic Therapy*, p. 119. (London: Churchill Livingstone)

80 Cumie, A. R. W. and Rachmaninoff, N. (1965). Fungal (candida) endocarditis following open heart surgery. *J. Thoracic and Cardiovascular surgery*, **50**, 431

81 Leffert, R. L. and Hackett, R. L. (1967). Aspergillus aortitis following replacement of an aortic valve. *J. Thorac. Cardiovasc. Surg.*, **53**. 866

82 Conway, N., Kothari, M. L., Lockey, E. and Yacoub, M. H. (1968). Candida endocarditis after heart surgery. *Thorax*, **23**, 353

83 Jones, T., Meshel, L. and Rubin, I. L. (1969). Aspergillus endocarditis superimposed on aortic valve prosthesis. *N. Y. State J. Med.*, **69**, 1923

84 Chaudhury, M. R. (1970). Fungal endocarditis after valve replacements. *J. Thorac. Cardiovasc. Surg.*, **60**, 207

85 Leading Article. (1975). Candida endocarditis. *Brit. Med. J.*, **2**, 264

86 Turnier, E., Kay, J. K., Bernstein, S., Mendez, A. M. and Zabiate, P. (1975). Surgical treatment of candida endocarditis. *Chest*, **67**, 262

87 Record, C. O., Skinner, J. M., Sleight, P. and Speller, D. C. E. (1971). Candida endocarditis treated with 5-fluorocytosine. *Brit. Med. J.*, **1**, 262

88 Darrell, J. H. (1975). Candida endocarditis. *Brit. Med. J.*, **1**, 432

89 Raper, A. J. and Kemp, V. E. (1965). Use of steroids in penicillin-sensitive patients with bacterial endocarditis. *N. Engl. J. Med.*, **279**, 1305

90 Green, G. R., Peters, G. A. and Geraci, J. E. (1967). Treatment of bacterial endocarditis in patients with penicillin hypersensitivity. *Ann. Intern. Med.*, **67**, 235

91 Assem, E. S. K. and Vickers, M. R. (1974). Penicillin allergy tests in man. *Immunology*, **27**, 255

92 Rahal, J. J., Myers, B. R. and Weinstein, L. (1968). Treatment of bacterial endocarditis with cephalothin. *N. Engl. J. Med.*, **279**, 1305

93 Fekety, F. R. and Weiss, P. (1966). Antibiotic synergism: Enhanced susceptibility of enterococci to combinations of streptomycin and penicillin or cephalosporins. *Antimicrob. Agents Chemother.*, **6**, 156

94 Durack, D. T., Starkebaum, M. K., and Petersdorf, R. G. (1977). Chemotherapy of experimental streptococcal endocarditis. VI. Prevention of enterococcal endocarditis. *J. Lab. Clin. Med.*, **90**, 171

95 Mandell, G. L. (1976). Enterococcal endocarditis. In D. Kaye (ed.) *Infective Endocarditis*, p. 107. (Baltimore: University Park Press)

96 Friedberg, C. K., Rosen, K. M. and Bienstock, P. A. (1968). Vancomycin therapy for enterococcal and *Streptococcus viridans* endocarditis. *Arch. Int. Med.*, **122**, 134

97 Westenfelder, G. O., Paterson, P. Y., Reisberg, B. E. *et al.* (1973). Vancomycin-streptomycin synergism in enterococcal endocarditis. *J. Am. Med. Assoc.*, **223**, 37

98 Quinn, E. L., Pohlod, D., Madhavan, K., Burch, K., Fisher, E. and Cox, F. (1973). Clinical experience with cephazolin and other cephalosporins in bacterial endocarditis. *J. Infect. Dis.*, **128** (Suppl.), 5386

99 Rahal, J. J., Myers, B. R. and Weinstein, C. (1968). Treatment of bacterial endocarditis with cephalothin. *N. Engl. J. Med.*, **279**, 1305

100 Smith, I. M. (1971). Cephalosporin therapy of staphylococcal infection in adults. *Postgrad. Med. J.*, **47** (Suppl.), 78

101 Fiala, M. and Kaushrik, V. (1978). Cephradine in the treatment of infective endocarditis compared with cephazolin. In *Current Chemotherapy*. Proceedings of the 10th International Congress of Chemotherapy, Zurich, September 1977, **2**, 867–869

102 Braimbridge, M. (1973). Surgery for bacterial endocarditis of heart valves. In A. M.

Geddes and J. D. Williams (eds.) *Current Antibiotic Therapy*. (Edinburgh: Churchill Livingstone)

103 English, T. A. H. and Ross, J. K. (1972). Surgical aspects of bacterial endocarditis. *Brit. Med. J.*, **4**, 598

104 American Heart Association Committee Report (1977). Prevention of bacterial endocarditis. *Circulation*, **56**, 139A

105 Hilson, G. F. R. (1970). Is chemoprophylaxis necessary? *Proc. R. Soc. Med.*, **63**, 267

106 Durack, D. T. and Petersdorf, R. G. (1973). Chemotherapy of experimental streptococcal endocarditis. Comparison of commonly recommended prophylactic regimes. *J. Clin. Invest.*, **52**, 592

107 Pelletier, L. L., Durack, D. T. and Petersdorf, R. G. (1975). Chemotherapy of experimental streptococcal endocarditis. IV. Further observations on prophylaxis. *J. Clin. Invest.*, **56**, 319

108 Garrod, L. P. and Waterworth, P. M. (1962). The risks of dental extraction during penicillin treatment. *Brit. Heart J.*, **24**, 39

109 Sewell, J. and Klar, S. (1975). Antibiotic cover for dental extractions. *Brit. Med. J.*, **3**, 540

110 Leading Article. (1975). Antibiotic cover for dental extractions. *Brit. Med. J.*, **3**, 191

111 Shanson, D. C. (1978). Infections of the heart. *Medicine*, **4**, 201

112 Shanson, D. C. (1978). The prophylaxis of infective endocarditis. *J. Antimicrob. Chemother.*, **4**, 2

113 Shanson, D. C., Cannon, P. and Wilks, M. (1978). Amoxycillin compared with penicillin V for the prophylaxis of dental bacteraemia. *J. Antimicrob. Chemother.*, **4**, 431

114 Shanson, D. C., Ashford, R. F. U. and Singh, J. (1979). Serum amoxycillin levels following 3.0 and 4.0 gram doses of amoxycillin. (In preparation)

115 Johnson, W. P., Cobbs, C. G., Arditti, C. S. and Kaye, D. (1968). Diphtheroid endocarditis after insertion of prosthetic heart valve. *J. Am. Med. Assoc.*, **203**, 919

116 Newsom, S. W. B. (1978). Antibiotic prophylaxis for open heart surgery. (Leading article). *J. Antimicrob. Chemother.*, **4**, 389

117 Nager, F., Pfisterer, M., Rothlin, R. and Kappenberger, L. (1975). Epidemiologie unk Klinik der Infektiosen Endokarditis. *Schweiz. Med. Wochenschr.*, **105**, 1421

118 Smith, R. H., Radford, D. J., Clark, R. A. and Julian, D. G. (1976). Infective endocarditis: A survey of cases in the South East region of Scotland, 1969–72. *Thorax*, **31**, 373

119 Shinebourne, E. A., Cripps, C. M., Hayward, G. W. and Shooter, R. A. (1969). Bacterial endocarditis 1956–65: analysis of clinical features and treatment in relation to mortality. *Brit. Heart J.*, **31**, 536

120 Johnson, R. H. *et al.* (1977). *Haemophilus endocarditis:* new cases literature review and recommendations for management. *South. Med. J.*, **70**, 1098

121 Slaughter, L., Morris, J. E. and Starr, A. (1973). Prosthetic valvular endocarditis. *Circulation*, **47**, 1319

122 Conway, N. (1969). Endocarditis in heroin addicts. *Brit. Heart J.*, **31**, 543

123 Ramsey, R. G., Gunnar, R. M. and Tobin, J. R. (1970). Endocarditis in the drug addict. *Am. J. Cardiol.*, **25**, 608

124 Banks, T., Fletcher, R. and Ali, N. (1973). Infective endocarditis in heroin addicts. *Am. J. Med.*, **55**, 444

125 Stimmel, B., Donoso, E. and Dack, S. (1973). Comparison of infective endocarditis in drug addicts and non-drug users. *Am. J. Cardiol.*, **32**, 924

126 Curtis, J., Richman, B. L., and Feinstein, M. A. (1974). Infective endocarditis in drug addicts. *South Med. J.*, **67,** 4
127 Cannon, N. J. and Cobbs, C. G. (1976). Infective endocarditis in drug addicts. In D. Kaye (ed.) *Infective Endocarditis.* (Baltimore: University Park Press)
128 Stokes, E. J. (1975). *Clinical Bacteriology,* 4th ed. (London: Arnold)
129 Colman, G. and Williams, R. E. (1972). Taxonomy of some human viridans streptococci. In C. W. Wannamaker and J. M. Mattsen (eds.) *Streptococci and Streptococcal Diseases; Recognition, Understanding and Management,* p. 281. (New York and London)
130 Hardie, J. M. and Bowden, G. H. (1976). Physiological classification of oral viridans streptococci. *J. Dent. Res.,* **55** (Special issue), A166

2

Prophylactic antimicrobial drug therapy

M. W. Casewell

INTRODUCTION

Most clinicians are from time to time perplexed about what can and cannot be achieved by prophylactic antimicrobial therapy. Few topics in therapeutics have generated such confusion, controversy, and heated debate.

Despite the arguments there seems to be one consensus, namely that antimicrobial prophylaxis is over-used. The disastrous consequences of infection on the one hand (for example in total hip replacements), and the availability and diversity of apparently effective antibiotics on the other, has too readily tempted the clinician into misguided prescription of prophylactic antimicrobial drug therapy. Prophylaxis, as George Bernard Shaw said of marriage, seems to be "popular because it combines the maximum of temptation with the maximum of opportunity"[1].

Accurate information about the prescribing habits of clinicians is not easy to find, but a recent review of antibiotic usage in North America[2] revealed that a quarter to a third of all patients in general wards received antibiotics. The indication for about half these prescriptions was "prophylaxis". A survey of prophylactic therapy in five London teaching hospitals[3] (which were discreetly not identified, the article being headed "Questionable Routines") revealed a diversity of curious regimens employed in these otherwise reputable centres.

The hope that antibacterial agents would ultimately abolish bacteria as a cause of serious infection and death has overtly not been realised. In

33

particular there remains a residue of hospital-acquired infection, often caused by Gram-negative bacilli or anaerobic bacteria, which threatens otherwise successful modern medical and surgical procedures. The enthusiasm to prevent these infections with antibiotics has not always been tempered by the constraints of rational scientifically based medicine. The literature abounds with conflicting views on a multiplicity of chemoprophylactic regimens, most of which have had only a cursory evaluation for efficacy and side-effects. Probably no other group of pharmacological agents has been so often prescribed on the basis of inadequate evidence and the clinician's idiosyncratic preference.

Thus, it is opportune to look again at the general principles and essential features of rational prophylaxis. Reiteration of these should help clarify our interpretation of published evidence that favours particular regimens and help define the absolute and provisional indications for chemoprophylaxis. With less dogma and a few more open verdicts it should be possible to identify those indications that still need further evaluation and those uses that are totally unfounded. A move towards accepting only rational regimens which are also supported by the results of controlled trials would substantially improve patient care.

What is chemoprophylaxis?
There are difficulties about a generally accepted definition of chemoprophylaxis. The administration of antibiotics for a short time before inoculation is an ideal approach for successful prevention of clinical infection, and few would doubt that this constitutes chemoprophylaxis. However, the administration of antibiotics *after* inoculation but *before* the onset of clinical infection is more problematic. Should this use of antibiotics be regarded as 'treatment' of the bacterial inoculum or 'prophylaxis' of clinical infection? As we are primarily concerned with preventing clinical infection it is this end-result which should be central in the definition of prophylaxis, i.e. *the administration of antimicrobial agent(s) before, or soon after, the inoculation of tissues in order to prevent the development of subsequent clinical infection.* Thus the use of sulphonamides for close domestic contacts of meningococcal disease may achieve one or more of these objectives, all of which constitute prophylaxis. The sulphonamides may protect siblings who are not yet nasopharyngeal carriers, they may eradicate the organism in established carriers (and prevent them subsequently developing clinical infection), and this elimination of carriers will prevent the spread of meningococci to susceptible contacts.

Doubts also arise about the distinction between treatment and prophylaxis when the antimicrobial agents are used in an attempt to prevent the extension of established infection to other sites. For example, does the perioperative administration of metronidazole at appendicectomy represent treatment of the appendicitis and the local peritonitis or prophylaxis of postoperative wound infection? Either is possible, but the intention should be clear, as the duration of the antibiotic courses for prophylaxis and treatment of the established infection may well be different.

ESSENTIAL FEATURES OF RATIONAL CHEMOPROPHYLAXIS

For any proposed regimen for antimicrobial prophylaxis there are five considerations that clarify the objectives and help assess the probability of success. What is the natural history of the infection in the absence of prophylaxis? Are there unexploited alternatives to antibiotics that might more effectively decrease the infection rate? Which antibiotic is to be used, and how should it be administered? Bearing in mind the documented claims that may already exist for success (and failure) for the proposed regimen, what are the chances of its success? Lastly, what are the undesirable unintended consequences of our attempts at potentially successful prophylaxis?

Infection in the absence of prophylaxis

Incidence
Unless the incidence of the particular infection is known it will be impossible to detect a decreased morbidity after the introduction of chemoprophylaxis. Furthermore, one is encouraged to devise prophylaxis for more common infections, such as wound sepsis following gastrointestinal surgery, or recurrent urinary tract infection. However, relatively infrequent infections such as endocarditis after heart valve replacement, which have such devastating consequences for a few patients, will also reinforce the need for effective prophylaxis.

Consequences of infection
Many infections are self-limiting or can be treated effectively with antibiotics, and although the morbidity and economic consequences of these cannot be dismissed, it is the infections with irreversible or life-threatening consequences that have rightly been given priority for chemoprophylaxis. For example, the desirability of preventing infection

of extensive burns, sepsis of surgical prostheses, bacterial endocarditis, and postoperative gangrene is self-evident.

Apart from individual patients in hospital, successful prophylaxis can have more subtle epidemiological benefits for the non-hospital community. For example, the control of outbreaks of meningococcal meningitis and diphtheria depend in part on the prophylactic treatment of close contacts of known cases.

In the enthusiasm to prevent infection it should be remembered that antibiotics are still of prime importance for the treatment of serious established infections. If these agents become effete because of the emergence of bacterial resistance following their exploitation for in-effective prophylaxis, then the outcome of many infections that at present can be adequately treated with antibiotics will be altered for the worse.

Timing of inoculation

Certain knowledge of the timing of inoculation is invaluable when one devises a rational regimen for antimicrobial prophylaxis, for this is when the antibiotic should be present at the site of inoculation for the first time, and not for hours or days before.

Sometimes one can be certain of this timing. For example, inoculation of the tissues in a deep wound infection, or of the blood in urological or cardiac surgery patients, commonly occurs in the theatre during the operative procedure. But often the timing of events is less predictable. Burns can become infected at any time after the thermal injury. The time of transmission of meningococci from a case or a carrier is unpredictable. The timing of the next streptococcal infection of a child with recurrent rheumatic fever cannot be known, and thus penicillin prophylaxis must be given until the child is adolescent and no longer at risk.

Causative bacteria

Prophylaxis is much more likely to be successful if one knows the bacteria, or at least the group of bacteria, that are likely to cause the infection that is to be prevented. Indeed, with this information it may be possible to preclude the necessity for prophylactic antibiotics altogether by taking measures that intercept the transmission of the organism to the site of inoculation. If prophylactic antibiotics do seem feasible, then an agent with the appropriate spectrum of activity can be selected. For example, the successful chemoprophylaxis of post-operative gas gangrene reflects our knowledge of the causative organism, *Clostridium perfringens,* and its predictable sensitivity to penicillin. We shall see later the confusion that can arise in the selection of chemoprophylactic agents when the causative organisms are not clearly recognised. For example many of the earlier attempts at preventing sepsis after large bowel surgery were confounded because the dominant role of non-sporing anaerobes was not appreciated.

Alternatives to antibiotics?

Even when the natural history of the infection is well known and prophylaxis seems possible, every effort should be made to ensure that established preventative measures, other than chemoprophylaxis, are being fully implemented.

Gilmore and his colleages have, for example, shown that instillation of interparietal povidone iodine at the end of abdominal operations reduced the incidence of postoperative wound infection.[4] The rationale is clear. This antiseptic has a broad spectrum of antibacterial activity, is non-toxic, and is placed where and when it is most needed to give high local concentrations. Hypersensitivity is not a problem, presumably because elemental iodine is not liberated, and resistant organisms do not emerge *in vitro* in series of povidone–iodine dilutions[5] or after prolonged clinical usage. It is remarkable how many surgeons are apparently unaware of the results of such controlled studies and prefer to continue to use various topical and systemic antibiotic regimens, most of which are of unproven value and may be actually harmful.

Historically there are many examples of improvements in nursing and surgical procedures that have contributed far more to the prevention of hospital-acquired infection than many attempts at antibiotic prophylaxis. The use of antibiotics some years ago in attempts to prevent bacteriuria in catheterised patients now seems naive when one considers the decrease in infection following the introduction of closed catheter drainage[6]. Some clinicians, at least in some London teaching hospitals[3], apparently still favour antibiotic 'prophylaxis' for their catheterised patients, and are undeterred by the lack of evidence that such regimens are of any value. Perhaps more scrupulous attention to catheter care and energetic supervision of nursing procedures might more effectively reduce the number of urinary tract infections.

Severely ill patients who require admission to intensive care, neonatal or burns units are particularly prone to colonisation and infection with Gram-negative bacilli, especially *Pseudomonas, Klebsiella,* and *Serratia* species. The use of *ad hoc* regimens of chemoprophylaxis in such patients may actually increase the infection rate[7] [8]. Our increasing knowledge of the epidemiology of these species is revealing important, but sometimes still neglected, sources for outbreaks of Gram-negative infection, including nebulisers and humidifiers, infusion fluids, ice-machines and anaesthetic equipment[9]. Ventilators are difficult to disinfect and still give rise to cross-infection with pseudomonas from time to time[10]. The epidemiology of endemic klebsiella and serratia infection has been more difficult to unravel, but the role of hands as a route of transmission for klebsiellae, and perhaps other Gram-negative bacilli, has probably been underestimated, and scrupulous handwashing by staff may prevent more klebsiella infection[11] than any amount of so-called antimicrobial prophylaxis[8].

Another approach to the prevention of Gram-negative infection is the use of vaccines. Workers in Birmingham have already had encouraging results with pseudomonas vaccine used for burned patients[12]. Uncontrolled hospital outbreaks with antibiotic-resistant klebsiellae[13] or serratia[14] may encourage the future development and use of vaccines to protect particularly vulnerable patients.

When all the alternatives have been fully deployed, there will remain certain infections for which antimicrobial prophylaxis seems both desirable and feasible.

Choice and administration of antibiotic

Spectrum
It is essential, of course, that the selected antibiotic should be active against the causative organism, but the overall antibacterial spectrum should be narrow so that there is minimal disturbance of the patient's normal flora. The prescription of several antibiotics in order to obtain a broad spectrum is no substitute for a knowledge of the likely causative bacteria and their sensitivity.

Toxicity
Once instituted, the routine use of a prophylactic regimen results in a massive increase in the overall consumption of that antimicrobial agent. Thus there will be a significant morbidity from even quite uncommon toxic side effects. A majority of those with drug toxicity would not have acquired the infection in the absence of prophylaxis. Thus toxicity must be carefully weighed against the potential benefits of successful prophylaxis.

Pharmacokinetics
Adequate concentrations of antibiotic should be present in the appropriate tissues at the time of inoculation. Pharmacokinetic considerations will thus influence the choice of agent, its dose, the route of administration, and the timing of the prophylactic doses. For example, low-dose cephalexin at bedtime can prevent recurrent cystitis because of its excretion, in active form, in the urine at the time of introduction of

bacteria into the bladder[15]. But maximum doses of parenteral gentamicin might be needed to give adequate blood levels in order to prevent bacteraemia in patients with bacteriuria who undergo urethral instrumentation. Although penicillin is active against meningococci it fails to reach adequate mucosal levels in the nasopharynx, and is thus unreliable for protecting non-carriers or treating the nasopharyngeal carriage of close domestic contacts of meningococcal disease.

Topical antibiotics
The principle of providing adequate local levels of antibiotic at the site of inoculation can be extrapolated to placing the antibiotic directly into surgical wounds on closure. For example, it has been shown that 1 g of cephaloridine used in this way significantly reduces the incidence of surgical wound infection[16]. The evidence favouring more exotic antibiotics is less convincing. There remain, however, serious doubts about the selection of resistant organisms when antibiotics are used in this way, especially when one considers the progressively falling local levels of antibiotic. The use of topical aminoglycosides has been clearly associated with the emergence of resistant organisms[17]. Also, unpredictable amounts of antibiotic may be absorbed, and the risk from toxicity is uncertain.

Timing of chemoprophylaxis
When, as in surgery, the timing of inoculation is known, the prophylactic antibiotic should be given for the first time just before the procedure, often with the pre-medication, so that the first peak serum level coincides with inoculation of the causative bacteria.

In the past there has been a tendency to start treatment too early and stop it too late. As recently as 1975 it was found that, whilst attempting to prevent endocarditis following tooth extraction in patients with damaged heart valves, as many as 38% of North American physicians started prophylaxis two days before the procedure[18]. Such premature treatment almost guarantees that the inevitable bacteraemia will be caused by penicillin-resistant organisms, and any subsequent endocarditis will be correspondingly difficult to treat. Similarly, prolonged preoperative chemoprophylaxis of patients who are to have gastrointestinal operations may only serve to replace antibiotic-sensitive gut flora with resistant strains.

In general, prophylaxis should be short, and 24 hours is often adequate. Fortunately, penicillin-resistant strains of β-haemolytic streptococci have not emerged in children who have received penicillin for many years for prophylaxis against recurrent attacks of rheumatic fever, an uncommon example of justifiably prolonged chemoprophylaxis necessitated by the unpredictability of subsequent streptococcal infection.

Does prophylaxis work?

Most of the controversy regarding chemoprophylaxis centres around
whether or not various regimens actually work, and it must be stressed
that it is impossible to assess the effectiveness of prophylaxis in
individual patients. Many variable factors, quite independent of antibiotics, affect rates of infection. In surgery for example, the patient's
pathology, the surgical procedure, the operator, the length of operation,
haemostasis, and the conditions in the operating theatre, may all
influence infection.

Thus we depend on the results of formal, carefully designed, properly
conducted, prospective, controlled clinical trials, and such trials are
feasible for infections with a moderate incidence. However, the
literature abounds with the results of small uncontrolled trials which do
not lend themselves to statistical evaluation, yet are often used by
clinicians as the basis for widespread antibiotic prescription. Some
would argue that editors of specialist journals have not always met their
responsibility for rejecting work that precipitates premature introduction of unproven regimens.

However, for uncommon infections, such as bacterial endocarditis or
infection of orthopaedic implants, it can be extremely difficult to design
trials that would detect a reduction in the already low incidence of
infection. For example, about 2500 observations under control conditions would be required to show a reduction in the incidence of
infection from 2% to 1%, with an 80% chance of demonstrating this
reduction at the 99% level of significance (or a 90% chance at the 95%
level). As one surgical team is most unlikely to perform the same
operation more than 200 or 300 times per year any trial of
chemoprophylaxis would have to be multicentered.

Even with results from well designed trials there are questions that
must be asked. Have all the variables been defined and where possible
controlled? What criteria have been used for diagnosing the infection?
Is the distinction between causative bacteria and laboratory isolates
clear? What was the quality of the bacteriology? If the laboratory cannot
isolate anaerobes then one cannot assess the anaerobic infection rate, with
or without chemoprophylaxis.

Even initially successful regimens will subsequently fail if, after
months or years, organisms emerge that are resistant to the prophylactic
antibiotic. Thus it is important to monitor prospectively the sensitivity
of the hospital flora. Pollock and Evans, for example, have shown that
despite the widespread use of prophylactic cephaloridine for general

surgical patients[19] an increase in cephaloridine-resistance of hospital strains was not detected some years later[20].

Undesirable consequences of chemoprophylaxis

Not only may prophylactic regimens fail to prevent infection, but they may generate new problems of toxicity and antimicrobial resistance.

The introduction of routine chemoprophylaxis results in a staggering increase in antibiotic consumption. For example, assume that an antibiotic is to be used for chemoprophylaxis in a group of patients for whom there is usually a 10% infection rate, and that hitherto only infected patients have been treated with this antibiotic. After the introduction of the prophylactic regimen, amongst every 100 patients receiving the antibiotic, there will be 90 who were not destined to be infected. This is equivalent to a 900% increase in the use of the antibiotic. The implications for toxic side-effects and the selective pressure favouring resistant bacteria are obvious.

In individual patients, the administration of antibiotics, for any purpose, sooner or later results in replacement of normal flora by antibiotic-resistant organisms which may then infect the patient himself, serve as a source for cross-infection of others, and ultimately contribute to the hospital environmental reservoir of resistant bacteria. Resistant strains may carry plasmids which, by conjugation, can transfer their resistance to other unrelated and previously sensitive species. Earlier suggestions that conjugation might be largely an *in vitro* phenomenon[21] are not supported by observations of conjugation in burns[22] and the urinary tract[23].

Apart from individual patients it is probable that the continued emergence of antibiotic-resistance amongst major pathogens reflects the ecological pressure of antibiotic use, more than half of which may be accounted for by chemoprophylaxis[2]. The implications for the non-hospital community in certain parts of the world are already serious. Chloramphenicol-resistant typhoid[24], haemophilus meningitis resistant to treatment with ampicillin[25], penicillin-resistant gonorrhoea[26], and most recently, pneumococcal meningitis no longer treatable with penicillin[27], are now a reality. In hospital-acquired infection, major epidemics of multiply-resistant *Klebsiella*[13] and *Serratia*[14] species are reported by an increasing number of hospitals throughout the world, and threaten the success of many modern medical and surgical procedures.

Thus the need to halt the massive antibiotic consumption for prophylaxis of uncertain value is clear. It is, however, more difficult to know how readily we should introduce new prophylactic regimens of *proven* efficacy on a routine basis. The value of reducing morbidity and mortality from infection is obvious, but this must be balanced against the possible future loss of further agents that are at present effective for treating established infection. It may be that the ability of micro-organisms to acquire resistance may yet outpace the pharmaceutical industry's capacity to discover, market, and conserve new effective antimicrobial agents.

ABSOLUTE AND PROVISIONAL INDICATIONS FOR CHEMOPROPHYLAXIS

The present widespread use of antibiotics for prophylaxis is often haphazard. However, attention to the essential features of rational prophylaxis outlined above, together with the results of clinical trials and other more indirect evidence, helps identify those conditions for which specific chemoprophylactic regimens almost certainly work and are generally considered to be mandatory. Common to all these indications is a knowledge of the organisms that cause the infection to be prevented. The antibiotic selected is directed specifically at these bacteria at the likely time of inoculation. Clinical trials of new regimens may in future enable us to extend these indications.

Rheumatic fever

Recurrences of rheumatic fever can be prevented by chemoprophylaxis directed against recurrent infection with *Streptococcus pyogenes*[28]. As the timing of inoculation with streptococci is unpredictable, prophylaxis must be prolonged. When the first episode is in childhood, prophylaxis should continue until the age of 17 or 18, or for at least 5 years, whichever is the longer[29]. It has been suggested[30] that more prolonged prophylaxis is required for those with heart damage, or for those admitted to hospital or entering an institution or camp, when there is a greater risk of exposure to streptococci. Adults with rheumatic fever should also continue prophylaxis for at least 5 years.

Sulphadiazine was initially used for prophylaxis of rheumatic fever, but its extensive use in the United States Armed Forces led to the emergence of sulphonamide-resistant streptococci[31]. However, penicillin is reliably bactericidal for *Str. pyogenes*, has a relatively narrow spectrum of activity, and is acceptably free of side-effects.

One thorough trial compared oral penicillin G (200 000 units once daily), intramuscular benzathine penicillin (1.2 mega units once monthly), and oral sulphadiazine (1 g per day)[28]. Benzathine penicillin most successfully prevented streptococcal infection, and only 6.1 streptococcal infections and 0.4 recurrences of rheumatic fever occurred per 100 patient years. The disadvantages of benzathine penicillin are the inconvenience of long-term intramuscular injections, and the possibility that any hypersensitivity reactions will be prolonged. For oral chemoprophylaxis the (British) Ministry of Health recommended[30] phenoxymethyl penicillin 125 mg twice daily, or penicillin G 200 000 units twice daily. Penicillin G is a curious choice as it is well known that it is not acid stable and is irregularly absorbed. Phenoxymethyl penicillin is probably the most widely used agent in the U.K. For patients who are hypersensitive to penicillin, oral sulphadimidine (0.5–1.0 g daily) was recommended.

Bacterial endocarditis
Patients with valvular heart disease or intracardiac prostheses are in danger of developing bacterial endocarditis following surgical procedures that are associated with bacteraemia. Dental manipulations, such as tooth extraction and the removal of stitches from the gums, and tonsillectomy are the commonest causes, although genito-urinary manipulations and bowel surgery may also result in bacteraemia. However, the actual risk for individual patients must be small, as less than a quarter of those with endocarditis give a history of dental manipulation and some may even be edentulous. Nevertheless the consequences of endocarditis are so serious that prevention of these few cases seems well worthwhile.

Bacterial endocarditis is most commonly caused by streptococci collectively known as the 'viridans' group, especially *Str. sanguis*, *Str. mutans*, *Str. mitior*, and *Str. milleri*. These oral streptococci, with various anaerobic bacteria, are indeed found in the blood of patients immediately after tooth extraction[33] [34]. In the past, uncertainties about the sensitivity of certain streptococci and other mouth organisms led some to believe that broad spectrum antibiotics, which were sometimes only bacteriostatic, might be useful. It is now clear that a bactericidal agent is required.

Few antibiotics can compare with the penicillin group for relative freedom from side-effects and bactericidal activity against oral streptococci, although it should be remembered that not all streptococci isolated from the blood after dental clearance are sensitive to penicillin[32].

The objective is to obtain bactericidal serum levels that coincide with the bacteraemia and are sustained for an adequate, although not excessive, postoperative period. Attempts to 'sterilise' the oropharynx with several days of preoperative antibiotic therapy are self-defeating, as the penicillin-sensitive flora is replaced by resistant bacteria which may then give rise to antibiotic-resistant endocarditis.

The rarity and seriousness of endocarditis have made it impossible to design ethical controlled trials to evaluate the efficacy of various regimens. Indirect evidence has been derived from studies on the bacteraemia following tooth extraction[33] and from the protective effect of certain antibiotics in animal experiments.

Durack and Petersdorf devised a rabbit model in which artificially damaged valves could be infected with streptococci, and the ability of various antibiotic regimens to prevent infection of the valves compared[34]. Tetracycline was ineffective, but a large dose of penicillin alone was successful provided adequate levels were sustained for 6–9 h after the bacteraemia. A single dose of vancomycin, or penicillin plus streptomycin, was effective. On the basis of these results the American Heart Association has favoured parenteral regimens which were often continued for 2 days. In 1977, for susceptible patients who do not have prosthetic valves (in whom endocarditis has a particularly poor prognosis), the revised recommendations included 1.0 mega unit of penicillin G intramuscularly plus 600 000 units intramuscularly 30 minutes before the procedure, followed by 500 mg penicillin V 6-hourly for eight doses. Intravenous vancomycin plus eight doses of erythromycin was recommended for penicillin hypersensitive patients.

These regimens have been criticised by Petersdorf[35] because of the obvious difficulty of giving injections to non-hospital patients and because the duration of therapy seemed excessive; he considers, as do others, that for adults 2 g of penicillin V given orally under supervision one hour before dental extraction followed by 500 mg orally 6-hourly for 24 hours is adequate. Shanson *et al.*[33], acknowledging the good anti-streptococcal activity, absorption, and prolonged serum activity of amoxycillin, have recently provided evidence that supports a single 2 g dose of oral amoxycillin given under supervision one hour before the dental extraction. This gives high serum levels in the following 6–8 h, which was considered critical in the rabbit model. For susceptible patients who are hypersensitive to penicillin 1 g oral erythromycin given half an hour before the procedure, followed by 500 mg orally every 8 h for three further doses, is acceptable[35]. Vancomycin, 1 g intravenously one hour before the procedure, as recommended by the American Heart Association, may well be more reliable.

Parenteral prophylaxis will still be required when endocarditis due to *Str. faecalis* following genito-urinary or lower bowel manipulations is to be prevented. Intramuscular or intravenous penicillin G (2 mega units) or ampicillin (1 g), plus intramuscular streptomycin (1 g) or intramuscular or intravenous gentamicin (maximum 80 mg) is suggested[35]. These should be given before the procedure and for two more doses afterwards, the intervals between the aminoglycoside doses being adjusted according to renal function.

Bacterial endocarditis is also a serious but uncommon complication of cardiac surgery, and the role of chemoprophylaxis is not known for certain. It is again difficult to envisage an adequate yet ethical controlled trial. About ten years ago the incidence of postoperative endocarditis was approximately 1%, but when intracardiac prostheses became generally available this rate went up to about 3–4%. Various 'prophylactic' regimens were subsequently devised and the infection rates reported. Sometimes the antibiotics were given for several days preoperatively, and sometimes only postoperatively. Many of the agents used were not effective against β-lactamase producing staphylococci, which were subsequently recognised as the major cause of postoperative intracardiac infection. In a useful review Phillips and Eykyn[36] noted that when β-lactamase antibiotics became available and were used for a short time preoperatively, and for an adequate time postoperatively, there was an associated fall in the published infection rates to less than 1%. Furthermore, the literature indicated that the proportion of staphylococci amongst the infecting bacteria fell from 63% to 24%. It is possible that these lowered infection rates merely reflected other improvements in surgical technique and practice, but today it is understandably difficult to convince a surgeon to abandon perioperative prophylaxis when he achieves an infection rate of less than 1%, and most would consider that chemoprophylaxis for cardiac surgery must be continued on an unproven but rational basis.

Many infections in open-heart surgery are caused by *Staphylococcus aureus* or *Staph. epidermidis,* but a few have been due to Gram-negative bacilli. The organisms are probably skin-derived and are inoculated at operation. The choice of antibiotics for prophylaxis has been recently reviewed by Newsom[37]. *Staph. epidermidis* has an unpredictable sensitivity and is often resistant to methicillin (and therefore cloxacillin and flucloxacillin) which would be predictably effective against *Staph. aureus.* Interestingly, the use of prophylactic anti-staphylococcal antibiotics does not seem to have resulted in an increase in postoperative endocarditis caused by Gram-negative bacilli or fungi, although there may be an increased isolation rate of Gram-negative bacilli from other sites.

Intramuscular cloxacillin or flucloxacillin with the premedication is commonly prescribed in the U.K., and 500 mg of flucloxacillin should probably be given intramuscularly for at least 2 days postoperatively; some continue for 5 days, but there is no evidence that this is any better than 2 days. The inclusion of gentamicin in the prophylaxis has the advantage of a spectrum that may include cloxacillin-resistant *Staph. epidermidis,* but it also causes a greater disturbance of the patient's normal flora, and may thus promote emergence of infection with gentamicin-resistant organisms in the postoperative period or later.

At Papworth hospital[37] the regimen consists of a loading dose, with the premedication, of cloxacillin, benzylpenicillin and gentamicin, given by intramuscular injection, followed by an intravenous booster at the end of the cardiopulmonary bypass to provide maximum levels as the operation finishes. Over the next 48 h, 1 mega unit of penicillin plus 500 mg cloxacillin, and gentamicin (according to age, weight and renal function), are given as an intravenous infusion. With this chemoprophylactic regimen there has been no case of prosthetic valve endocarditis in any of 800 open-heart operations at Papworth. Should there be a continued increase in gentamicin-resistant staphylococci and enterobacteria such a regimen will require revision.

Vancomycin or clindamycin seem to be rational choices for patients who are hypersensitive to penicillin. Another possibility is a cephalosporin, but the one selected should have a good stability to staphylococcal β-lactamase.

Readers interested in a review of the chemoprophylaxis of infective endocarditis should read the previous Chapter by Dr D. C. Shanson.

Postoperative gas gangrene

Gas gangrene is classically associated with traumatic dirty injuries or with bowel operations. More rarely, however, severe and often fatal sepsis with *Cl. perfringens (Cl. welchii)* may follow relatively clean surgery of the lower limb. The clostridia are probably derived from the patient's faecal flora, rather than the environment, and are implanted at operation into ischaemic tissue. Although preoperative skin preparation with povidone iodine may reduce the contaminating skin clostridia by about 90%, skin disinfection alone is not an adequate safeguard and prophylactic chemotherapy is now considered to be essential for amputation of ischaemia limbs[38].

Cl. perfringens is invariably sensitive to penicillin, and this seems to be a rational choice of antibiotic, but the rarity of this infection has made it difficult to design a controlled trial to test the efficacy of penicillin. However, in 1969, Parker[39] at the Central Public Health Laboratory, Colindale received notification of 56 cases of postoperative gas gangrene, 31 of which were fatal. He found that this infection most commonly followed amputation of the lower limb (39 out of 56) in elderly patients, and in almost all of these the indication for surgery was arterial insufficiency. Ten patients had diabetes, and 11 had had operations in the neighbourhood of the hip. One of the most important findings was that none of the patients who developed clostridial sepsis was being treated with adequate doses of penicillin on the day of operation.

The dose of penicillin usually recommended is 500 000 units of penicillin G intramuscularly, starting with the premedication and continuing for 5–7 days postoperatively. Some surgeons give 1 mega unit intramuscularly 6-hourly, as this is the largest dose that most patients can tolerate by this route. Tetracycline is not a substitute for penicillin, as tetracycline-resistant strains of *Cl. perfringens* have been found. For patients who are hypersensitive to penicillin Parker[39] recommended erythromycin as antibiotic of second choice. I have, however, seen one case of gas gangrene following the prophylactic use of intramuscular erythromycin. If erythromycin is used adequate levels should be ensured, and 600 mg intravenous erythromycin lactobionate should be given as an infusion over 5 minutes with the premedication and repeated (1–2 g per day, in divided doses) for five days postoperatively. Prophylactic metronidazole, or possibly clindamycin, which are active against *Cl. perfringens*, might be alternatives to penicillin for hypersensitive patients, but there is little evidence to prove their efficacy, and clyndamicin is associated with pseudomembranous colitis.

Meningococcal infections
Epidemic meningococcal infection occurs in institutions, such as military establishments, and amongst the close domestic contacts of a case of meningococcal disease, especially where there is overcrowded shared sleeping accommodation. A high rate of nasopharyngeal carriage often precedes the presentation of clinical cases, and those who fail to achieve a harmless carrier state acquire the disease – a concept known as 'failure of carriage'. Normal nasopharyngeal carriage rates are found in school contacts, and it is the very young close domestic contacts who are most at risk.

It is now well established that chemoprophylaxis given to these close contacts will eliminate the nasopharyngeal carriage and protect the vulnerable non-carriers. In England the majority of infections are caused by Group B strains, at least 80% of which are still fully sensitive to sulphadiazine which is the prophylactic antibiotic of choice. It should be given in full dosage (for adults, 1 g orally three times a day for 3 days), without waiting for the results of nasopharyngeal cultures. Sul-phadimidine is preferred by some, because of its increased solubility, but it has significantly less *in vitro* activity against meningococci. Penicillin fails to clear the nasopharynx[40] and should not be used.

More than half of Group A and an increasing number of B, C and W135 strains may be sulphonamide resistant[41] and the choice of prophylaxis for resistant strains is problematic. Oral rifampicin (600 mg daily for 4 days) reduces the carriage rate, but resistant strains soon emerge[42]. Minocycline has been used with some success[43], but vestibular side-effects have been reported in a large proportion of patients taking this drug[44]. At present rifampicin seems to be the only possible antibiotic for prophylaxis of sulphonamide-resistant meningococcal infection, but many consider that it should be restricted to the treatment of tuberculosis.

Diphtheria

The control of diphtheria outbreaks depends mostly on the isolation and treatment of cases, and the active immunisation of contacts with toxoid. Nevertheless, an appropriate antibiotic is prescribed to clear *Corynebacterium diphtheriae* from the nasopharynx of carriers, and this may help protect susceptible contacts whilst they are acquiring active immunity.

Most physicians consider that erythromycin is the drug of choice; it was effective as a 10–14 day course during the Manchester diphtheria outbreak in 1971, and there was no reversion to a carrier state over the following 6 months[45]. McCloskey *et al.*[46] found a single intramuscular injection of benzathine penicillin (600 000 units) in children aged 1–5 years as effective as oral erythromycin estolate given to children and adults (adult dose 250 mg four times a day for 7 days)[46].

Extensive burns

Infection remains the most important complication of extensive burns, and is the commonest cause of death. *Str. pyogenes, Staph. aureus,* and *Ps. aeruginosa* are the bacteria most commonly implicated, and specific systemic antimicrobial prophylaxis against *Str. pyogenes* is probably indicated for burns that exceed 10% of body surface area.

Formal proof of the efficacy of systemic penicillin G (1 mega unit 6-hourly for 5 days) is lacking but its reliable activity against streptococci (and against *Cl. tetani*), the frequency of serious streptococcal infection in the absence of prophylaxis, and the narrow spectrum of penicillin, make this a rational choice which many would consider essential[47]. Others have used erythromycin 250 mg 6-hourly, or cloxacillin 250 mg 6-hourly. Broad spectrum antibiotics are not a substitute, and these should be withheld until there is clinical or bacteriological evidence of infection (which is difficult to assess in burned patients) or positive blood cultures.

The role of topical prophylactic antibiotics and antiseptics is sometimes difficult to assess. The Birmingham group showed in a controlled trial[48] that compresses kept continuously moist with 0.5% silver-nitrate solution gave better protection against bacterial colonisation than a daily application of 11.2% mafenide ('Sulfamylon') acetate cream with exposure of burns, but infection with *Ps. aeruginosa* was similar. Both these methods were better than simply allowing the burns to be exposed to warm dry air at 30–32 °C. An improvement in mortality was not demonstrated. Disadvantages of silver-nitrate applications include electrolyte loss and staining of linen and fabrics.

Prosthetic implants in orthopaedic surgery
The dramatic advances following the use of orthopaedic prosthetic implants, such as total hip replacement, are still blighted by uncommon postoperative infections that usually result in the total failure of the operative procedure. Despite an extensive and often anecdotal surgical literature the role of antimicrobial prophylaxis is still not established, although most surgeons in the United Kingdom prefer to use it. There are also conflicting views regarding the value of topical antibiotics placed directly into the wound or incorporated in the acrylic bone cement. These problems will be discussed here in relation to total hip replacement, but many of the issues are similar for other prosthetic implants and for open fractures.

Infections of orthopaedic wounds are conventionally classified as superficial or deep, and for prosthetic implants it is the latter that are so destructive. In the absence of chemoprophylaxis the reported incidence may vary between 11% and less than 1%[49], but most surgeons have rates of less than 3%.

Renowned groups, such as that of Charnley and his colleagues at Wrightington Hospital, have achieved remarkably low sepsis rates without the use of systemic or topical chemoprophylaxis[50]. Others with higher rates, still wonder whether chemoprophylaxis would help and are uncertain about the relative contributions of ultra-clean air, surgical technique, and meticulous attention to asepsis. With low sepsis rates, any controlled trial to evaluate the contributory factors requires a large number of operations and must be multicentred. One such trial is continuing now in 17 UK centres and in Scandinavia.

The timing of inoculation is likely to be at operation, when organisms derived from the flora of the patient or theatre staff may be inoculated into the wound directly, or indirectly via the theatre air. Delayed sepsis sometimes occurs several months after the operation, when it has been suggested that bacteraemic spread occurs from some other, unidentified, source.

The causative organisms most commonly implicated are *Staph. aureus* and *Staph. epidermidis*[51]. However, a wide range of other isolates, including Gram-negative bacilli, have been reported but there is often a conspicuous failure to discriminate between the bacteria causing deep infection and those isolates representing secondary bacterial colonisation of an infected surface. For example, specimens taken from wounds during antibiotic therapy are more likely to reflect colonisation with opportunistic hospital-acquired Gram-negative bacilli. On the basis of the present evidence it seems clear that any prophylactic antibiotics should be directed primarily at *Staph. aureus.*

Assuming that antibiotics might decrease the infection rate, which antibiotic should be used? How should it be administered? Cloxacillin is active against most strains of *Staph. aureus,* but less predictable against *Staph. epidermidis.* It is bactericidal with a narrow spectrum of activity, and seems a rational choice. Ericson *et al.*[52], in one of the few controlled trials, had no infections in 83 patients given cloxacillin prophylaxis compared with 12 of 88 patients in the placebo group. The antibiotic group received 1 g of cloxacillin intramuscularly one hour before the operation and thereafter three further doses at 6-hourly intervals. This was followed by oral administration of 1 g 6-hourly until the 14th postoperative day. Each patient also received 1 g probenecid, orally twice a day.

The newer β-lactamase-stable penicillin, flucoxacillin, seems to be a suitable alternative; it is better absorbed, and significant amounts of active agent are found in bone samples taken at operation[53]. Although cephaloridine[54] and cefuroxime[55] have also been found in operative samples of bone and synovial capsule there remain doubts about the contribution of antibiotic in the contaminating blood. Furthermore, cephalosporins have an unnecessarily broad spectrum of activity, which will disturb the normal flora of the patient, and the instability of cephaloridine to staphylococcal β-lactamase is another theoretical disadvantage. Cefuroxime should for the present undoubtedly be reserved for treating established infections caused by Gram-negative bacilli which are resistant to most standard agents.

It is possible that infection occurring after the immediate postoperative period reflects blood-borne invasion of the joint from some other focus, rather than inoculation at operation. This has encouraged Buchholz to use an antibiotic incorporated in the bone cement so that diffusion of antibiotic in the surrounding tissues might protect against late bacterial complications. His impressive results (published in German) have been criticised on statistical and other grounds in a useful review on antibiotics in bone cement by Moore[56]. Overall, there remain more questions than answers, and on the basis of present evidence this should be regarded as an experimental procedure. For example, which antibiotic should be incorporated? How important is any weakening of the cement by incorporation of antibiotics? What are the kinetics of liberation of antibiotic from cement into the tissues of the patient? And how reliable are the results from experimental models? Does the delay in diffusion of the antibiotic produce a bactericidal concentration in the tissues at the time of operation? What are the risks of hypersensitivity for a drug that may be left in the body for many months? Are we confident that any hypersensitivity to the depot antibiotic will be recognised before the patient is challenged with the same antibiotic at some future date? With falling local concentrations of antibiotic, what chances are there of selecting resistant strains which may then infect the joint?

Finally, many orthopaedic surgeons confess to placing a fairly random selection of antibiotics into the wound at operation. The feeling that a local excess of antibiotic can only do good, may unfortunately not be true. In other contexts it is well known that topical agents may be associated with the hazards of toxicity, hypersensitivity and the emergence of resistant strains. The burden of proof remains with those who use these incompletely evaluated procedures.

Gastrointestinal and gynaecological surgery
Operations involving the opening of abdominal viscera may carry a 30% or even 50% postoperative infection rate. The enthusiasm to find the surgeon's utopia of 'surgery without sepsis' has generated a vast literature of conflicting results which were based on trials that were often poorly designed and uncontrolled. These reports have had wide influence on the prescription of antimicrobial agents.

In the past, three approaches have been explored, namely preoperative bowel preparation, topical agents placed into the wound, and systemic perioperative prophylaxis. The last of these has recently included new regimens based on secure bacteriological principles, and has been evaluated in convincing trials that show dramatic reductions in infection rates which constitute a significant advance in modern surgery.

Preoperative bowel preparation
Earlier preoccupations with producing a sterile bowel by preoperative non-absorbable oral agents now seem naive, especially as some of the recommended agents, such as neomycin, have no activity against the non-sporing anaerobes, now known to constitute at least 98% of the normal bowel flora[57] and to be one major cause of postoperative sepsis[58]. The warning 'if you want to sterilise the bowel, the only way to do it is to take it out and boil it'[59] has been particularly apt in view of present knowledge of anaerobes and their antibiotic sensitivities. Trials of

various oral agents on many thousands of patients have given no convincing consensus of efficacy. Indeed sometimes there is a suggestion that such regimens increase sepsis.

Potential harmful effects of such regimens include the disturbance of normal flora which may encourage staphylococcal enterocolitis, the suggestion of an increased risk of recurrent tumour in the suture line, and lastly, and most importantly, the emergence of bowel bacteria resistant to agents such as neomycin and more useful aminoglycosides. Even the value of preoperative mechanical cleansing of the colon by low residue diets, laxatives and bowel irrigation has been disputed[60], because the physical and antibacterial interference with the lumen might damage the colon's own mechanisms for defence against bacterial invasion.

Instillation of antimicrobial agents into the wound at operation
The instillation of antimicrobial agents directly into the wound at the end of the operation should give high local levels of antibiotic at the time of, or soon after, the inoculation of the wound with bowel organisms, but once again there are few prospective trials that are well controlled and randomised.

In Scarborough, Pollock, Evans and their colleagues have reported that instillation of 1 g of cephaloridine in 2 ml of water into the wound at closure is effective in reducing the wound sepsis rate in a variety of general surgical operations[16], and that this procedure was more effective than 0.5 g of topical framycetin[19]. Although there was a low isolation rate of anaerobic bacteria in the untreated controls it can be assumed that cephaloridine must have achieved a reduction in clinical anaerobic sepsis. Pollock and Evans used topical cephaloridine for more than three years, yet they were unable to detect an increase in cephaloridine resistance in Scarborough Hospital[20]. Nevertheless, the risk that resistance will emerge in future remains, and this regimen must now be judged in relation to more effective perioperative prophylaxis with agents that have a narrow antibacterial spectrum which have been successfully developed in the last few years.

The advantages of using a topical antiseptic, such as povidone iodine, in place of an antibiotic have already been mentioned in this Chapter. Despite the apparent efficacy of this agent[5], surgeons still often show a preference for haphazardly personal selected topical antibiotics of unproven efficacy.

Perioperative antibiotics
Many regimens have been devised that use systemic antibiotics administered at varying times around the time of operation. Care should be

taken to identify those patients who are already infected preoperatively, for in these the 'prophylactic' antibiotic also constitutes therapy.

Systemic antibiotics given for long periods before operation undoubtedly serve only to select resistant flora, and may even increase the infection rate. Prolonged postoperative prophylaxis also selects resistant strains and may delay the recognition of the infection it was meant to prevent.

One of the earliest controlled double-blind trials which restricted the antibiotic to the immediate preoperative period and a few doses postoperatively was that of Polk and Lopez-Meyer in 1969[61]. One gram of intramuscular cephaloridine given immediately before gastrointestinal operations, and two further doses 5 and 12 h later, was associated with an infection rate of 6% compared with 30% in the untreated control group. A measure of the dependence at that time on the clinical assessment of wounds is reflected by the complete absence of anaerobes in the recorded isolates from infected wounds.

Stokes *et al.*[62] in 1974, pointing out the importance of the anaerobic intestinal flora, utilised the activity of lincomycin against anaerobes by giving this agent with tobramycin (or gentamicin) immediately preoperatively and for only one dose postoperatively. Some overall success was recorded, but the diversity of operations, which ranged from splenectomy to hemicolectomy, made it impossible to assess the efficacy of the regimen for specified operative procedures.

Although aerobic coliforms are often isolated from anaerobic infections it is becoming clear that antimicrobial prophylaxis (or treatment) need only be directed at the anaerobic component of the infection. As *Bacteroides fragilis* is consistently sensitive only to clindamycin (or lincomycin), metronidazole, and probably cefoxitin, the rational choice of agents for prophylaxis is limited.

Remarkable results have been obtained by Willis and his many colleagues[63][64] at Luton and Dunstable Hospital in double-blind, prospective, well controlled trials which utilise the anaerobic activity of metronidazole. In appendicectomy patients 1 g metronidazole was given rectally in a suppository with the premedication and repeated 8-hourly until oral feeding began, when 200 mg of metronidazole was given orally three times a day until the end of the 7th postoperative day; anaerobic infection was reduced from 19 to zero per cent[63]. A similar regimen started 24 hours preoperatively (plus a single 80 mg preoperative dose of gentamicin) for elective colonic surgery gave no anaerobic infections compared to 58% in the untreated controls[64]. In hysterectomy patients, 2 g of oral metronidazole on admission followed by 200 mg orally three times a day until the 7th postoperative day reduced the anaerobic infection rate from 23 to one per cent[65].

Whether the routine use of metronidazole for these common operations will hasten the emergence of metronidazole-resistant anaerobes remains to be seen. With this reservation, it may well be improper to withold the metronidazole for chemoprophylaxis in these defined groups of patients.

The use of tobramycin, and even more valuable newer aminoglycosides, for prophylaxis should be recognised as unnecessary (*vide supra*) and particularly wasteful of aminoglycosides needed for treatment of infections with gentamicin-resistant Gram-negative bacilli, which may assume epidemic proportions[13].

The well-established association of lincomycin or clindamycin with pseudomembranous colitis[66] probably precludes the use of these agents as a substitute for metronidazole. In a trial[67] of 25 patients receiving lincomycin, six developed pseudomembranous colitis (three of whom had received only three doses each), and two actually died. One year later in a different hospital[68], of 14 patients given prophylactic lincomycin and gentamicin, two developed pseudomembranous colitis, and one died; to continue with the gentamicin/lincomycin combination was 'not thought to be advisable'. The well recognised sporadic nature of pseudomembranous colitis (possibly accounted for by the epidemiology of the causative bacterium *Cl. difficile*) might finally embarrass the last defenders of lincomycin for prophylactic use in patients with established gut disease (Griffiths *et al.* (1976)[69]; Galland *et al.* (1977)[70]), albeit for single dose or short courses.

In future it should be possible to ascertain whether the successful regimens with metronidazole can be shortened, perhaps to a single intravenous infusion, in defined patient groups, and whether metronidazole resistance will limit the continued use of effective prophylaxis.

Urological patients
Despite the lack of formal trials there is a rational case for chemoprophylaxis for certain urological procedures which are associated with bacteraemia caused by organisms derived from the urinary tract.

At St Thomas' Hospital we have recently defined the susceptible patients by examining the detailed clinical and bacteriological records of urological patients who, over a 10 year period, had bacteraemia[71]. Of 40 bacteraemias, 24 followed instrumentation and in 22 of these the urine was infected at the time of operation, and only one patient was receiving an appropriate antibiotic. Patients undergoing transrectal biopsy, difficult urethral dilatation or, less predictably, repeated urethral catheterisation, often had bacteraemia in the absence of bacteriuria. All but six of the blood isolates (usually enterobacteria, pseudomonas, or staphylococci) were sensitive to gentamicin.

Having defined the small group of patients who are at risk and the most likely bacteria involved, we now use perioperative gentamicin, 120 mg intramuscularly with the premedication, and two further doses of 80 mg at appropriate intervals postoperatively. If the sensitivity of the urine isolate is known, a rational agent is selected accordingly. Since the introduction of this policy there have been no bacteraemias in these groups of patients at risk.

Recurrent urinary tract infection

Recurrent symptomatic 'urinary tract infection' occurs most commonly in women of child-bearing age. About one half of these episodes are associated with bacteriuria, but the urinary tract is usually radiologically normal.

The association with sexual intercourse suggested that postcoital micturition may help prevent attacks, but where this fails low dose antimicrobial agents taken at night might prevent the organisms multiplying in the bladder. Controlled trails have shown that 50 mg nitrofurantoin[72] or 125 mg cephalexin[15] at night are both effective in this group of patients. Nitrofurantoin should not be given to women with inpaired renal function.

In a group of women and girls, with normal renal function, but unspecified radiological status, a regimen based on an adult dose of 40 mg trimethoprim and 200 mg sulphamethoxazole taken at bedtime was more effective than sulphamethoxazole alone, methenamine mandelate or no treatment[73]. Low dose co-trimoxazole given once a day to children, many of whom had abnormal intravenous pyelograms, was used in another trial which, although uncontrolled, produced a convincingly low recurrence rate[74].

The duration of low-dose prophylaxis in all these regimens is not clear and will have to be judged for individual patients.

Tuberculosis

'Chemoprophylaxis' of tuberculosis may refer to true prevention of the disease, prevention of the clinical disease in positive tuberculin reactors, prevention of relapse of apparently inactive disease, or treatment of cases and non-infected individuals in whole communities. These uses of prophylaxis cannot be considered in isolation, but this complex subject is beyond the scope of this review and the interested reader is therefore referred to a recent British Medical Journal editorial[75].

Malaria

The incidence of malaria imported into the UK is increasing. It most commonly occurs in those who fail to take appropriate prophylaxis, many of whom may be immigrants resident in the United Kingdom who are returning to a malarious zone. The choice of prophylactic drug depends on a knowledge of the malarious countries and whether chloroquine-resistant falciparum malaria is known. This information, together with appropriate regimens, is given in useful publications from the World Health Organisation[76] and the Center for Disease Control[77].

Prevention measures, such as screening of windows, aerosol sprays, mosquito netting and insect repellent, are important but in a malarious zone are not a substitute for chemoprophylaxis which is absolutely indicated for travellers from non-epidemic zones.

One of the antifolates is most commonly prescribed for travellers from Britain to areas which are endemic for chloroquine-sensitive strains. Proguanil (adult dose 100 mg daily, or 200 mg daily for tropical Africa), or pyrimethamine (adult dose 25–50 mg weekly) should be started the day before departure and continued for 8 weeks after returning from the malarious country. Chloroquine, a 4-aminoquinoline, which is useful for treatment of malaria, is not favoured by authorities in this country for chemoprophylaxis, because of the theoretical risk that its use in this way might accelerate the emergence of chloroquine-resistant plasmodia.

Because of cross-resistance between the 4-aminoquinolines and the antifolates, the antifolates are inappropriate for chemoprophylaxis for those visiting countries which have chloroquine-resistant malaria. A synergistic combination of pyrimethamine (25 mg) and sulfadoxine (500 mg)), 'Fansidar', is now recommended by WHO. One tablet of Fansidar every week is the normal adult dose, and no serious toxicity was found when the drug was taken for up to one year.

UNCERTAIN INDICATIONS FOR
CHEMOPROPHYLAXIS

Acute leukaemia and immune deficiency
Neutropenia is the most important contributing factor to the morbidity and mortality from infection in patients with acute leukaemia. The source of bacteria for septicaemic episodes is not always apparent, but, in the absence of antibiotic therapy, the commonest causative organisms are similar to those for septicaemia in other patients, and the more exotic opportunists are relatively infrequently implicated. The potential value of chemoprophylaxis is still uncertain, despite numerous trials which yet again have often been poorly controlled in small groups of patients. Two recent leading articles summarise the evidence succinctly[78] [79], and it will suffice to mention here some of the approaches that have been attempted.

Various non-absorbable oral antibiotics have been tried in order to suppress normal bowel flora. Some evidence suggests that both the antibiotics and a protective environment make a contribution to reducing infection. A mixture of framycetin, colistin and nystatin (FRACON) with topical chlorhexidine reduced the frequency of infection and infectious deaths of patients nursed in simple protective isolation, but did not improve the remission rate[80].

A wide variety of intravenous and absorbed prophylactic antibiotics have also been tried, sometimes in rotation, with and without a protected environment. Sometimes it is difficult to elucidate the contribution of higher anti-leukaemic drug dosage, and it is right to question the likely effect of all these chemoprophylactic regimens on the hospital flora in terms of resistance. Most recently co-trimoxazole alone has been used with some success[81], and such a relatively simple regimen has obvious attractions.

Many still regard the contribution of chemoprophylaxis as uncertain, and prefer to monitor their patients for early signs of infection and reserve antibiotics for the treatment of infective episodes with relatively sensitive organisms, as and when such episodes occur.

Intensive care and neonatal patients
The difficulties of diagnosing infection in these susceptible patients has often encouraged the use of arbitary chemoprophylaxis. However, the many disadvantages of this approach that have already been discussed should be heeded. In neurosurgical intensive care patients, for example, chemoprophylaxis actually *increased* the rate of infection[8]. The use of antibiotics should, in general, be directed at specific infections, rather than 'broad cover', even if the diagnosis is provisional.

Chronic bronchitis
Some limited success has been obtained in two approaches to preventing acute exacerbations in chronic bronchitics.

Long-term continuous prophylaxis with oxytetracycline during the winter months may reduce the number of exacerbations in those patients who normally have frequent attacks. However, this has no effect on the declining respiratory function, but there may be some improvement in the number of days lost from work. Co-trimoxazole may be a suitable alternative, as the trimethoprim component gives good levels in the sputum. Ampicillin or cephalexin give too much bowel disturbance and are not suitable for continuous use.

A more rewarding approach for intelligent patients is to provide prophylactic antibiotics (which can be rotated from attack to attack or winter to winter) which should be started by the patient at the first sign of a head or chest cold. Co-trimoxazole, tetracycline, amoxycillin or erythromycin are all reasonable choices.

Interested readers are referred to a recent review by Hughes[82] for a fuller consideration and further references to this subject.

CONCLUSIONS

It is hoped that this review has served to illustrate the approach that is required for rational prophylaxis, and has outlined the present major surgical and medical indications. Cessation of arbitrary chemo-prophylactic regimens that are not sound in theory nor supported by evidence of efficacy would immediately improve the quality of patient care.

In future there will doubtless emerge new suggestions for chemoprophylaxis. When the theory and clinical trials supporting these regimens have been examined more critically than in the past there will doubtless be new defined situations where it is clear that chemo-prophylaxis prevents infection. The controversy, however, will not stop there. For having shown that a particular regimen does result in less morbidity and mortality from infection, these advantages must be balanced against the possibility that generalised use of these regimens will result in the emergence of antibiotic resistance. The price one may then pay for successful prophylaxis will be the accelerated erosion of useful antimicrobial agents that hitherto had been of life-saving value in established infection.

The ultimate price of increasing the use of antibiotics in this way may hasten the day when the antibiotic era is regarded as a transitory period of merely a few decades in the long history of medicine, when antibiotics existed as a valuable therapeutic aid to the clinician and his patient.

References

1 Shaw, G. B. (1947). *Man and Superman. Maxims for Revolutionists*, p. 24. (London: Constable)
2 Simmons, H. E. and Stolley, P. D. (1974). This is medical progress? Trends and consequences of antibiotic use in the United States. *J. Am. Med. Assoc.*, **227**, 1023
3 Report by the study group on the use of antimicrobial drugs. (1977). Prophylactic antimicrobial drug therapy at five London teaching hospitals. *Lancet*, **1**, 1351
4 Editorial. (1976). Prophylactic povidone iodine. *Lancet*, **1**, 73
5 Gilmore, O. J. A. and Sanderson, P. J. (1975). Prophylactic interparietal povidone-iodine in abdominal surgery. *Brit. J. Surg.*, **62**, 792
6 Ansell, J. (1962). Some observations on catheter care. *J. Chron. Dis.*, **15**, 675
7 Petersdorf, R. G., Curtin, J. A., Hoeprich, P. D., Peeler, R. N. and Bennett, I. L.

(1957). A study of antibiotic prophylaxis in unconscious patients. *New Engl. J. Med.*, **257**, 1001

8   Price, D. J. E. and Sleigh, J. D. (1970). Control of infection due to Klebsiella aerogenes in a neurosurgical unit by withdrawal of all antibiotics. *Lancet*, **2**, 1213

9   Parker, M. T., Bassett, D. J. C. and Lowbury, E. J. L. (1971). Causes and prevention of sepsis due to Gram-negative bacteria. Common source outbreaks. *Proc. R. Soc. Med.*, **64**, 980

10 Phillips, I. and Spencer, G. (1965). Pseudomonas aeruginosa cross-infection due to contaminated respiratory apparatus. *Lancet*, **2**, 1325

11 Casewell, M. and Phillips, I. (1977). Hands as a route of transmission for Klebsiella species. *Brit. Med. J.*, **2**, 1315

12 Jones, R. J., Roe, E. A. and Gupta, J. L. (1978). Low mortality in burned patients in a pseudomonas vaccine trial. *Lancet*, **2**, 401

13 Curie, K., Speller, D. C. E., Simpson, R. A., Stephens, M. and Cooke, D. I. (1978). A hospital epidemic caused by a gentamicin-resistant *Klebsiella aerogenes. J. Hyg. (Camb.)*, **80**, 115

14 Stratford, B. C., Dixson, S., Clarke, B. G. and Stratford, B. F. (1978). Epidemic of hospital-acquired infection due to *Serratia marcescens:* report of 104 cases. *Current Chemotherapy.* Proceedings of the 10th International Congress of Chemotherapy, Vol. 1, p. 442. (Washington, DC: American Society for Microbiology)

15 Gower, P. E. (1975). The use of small doses of cephalexin (125 mg) in the management of recurrent urinary tract infection in women. *J. Antimicrob. Chemother.*, **1** (Suppl.), 93

16 Evans, C., Pollock, A. V. and Rosenbery, I. L. (1974). The reduction of surgical wound infections by topical cephaloridine: a controlled clinical trial. *Br. J. Surg.*, **61**, 133

17 Wyatt, T. D., Ferguson, W. P., Wilson, T. S. and McCormick, E. (1977). Gentamicin resistant *Staphylococcus aureus* associated with the use of topical gentamicin. *J. Antimicrob. Chemother.*, **3**, 213

18 Neu, H. C. and Howrey, S. P. (1975). Testing the physician's knowledge of antibiotic use. Self-assessment and learning via videotape. *New Eng. J. Med.*, **293**, 1291

19 Pollock, A. V. and Evans, M. (1975). The prophylaxis of surgical wound sepsis with cephaloridine – experiences in 2,491 general surgical operations and reporting a controlled clinical trial against framycetin. *J. Antimicrob. Chemother.*, **1**, (Suppl.), 71 71

20 Pollock, A. V. and Evans, M. (1975). Changing patterns of bacterial resistance in relation to prophylactic use of cephaloridine and therapeutic use of ampicillin. *Lancet*, **2**, 1251

21 Lacey, R. W. (1975). A critical appraisal of the importance of R-factors in the enterobacteriaceae *in vivo. J. Antimicrob. Chemother.*, **1**, 25

22 Roe, E. and Jones, R. J. (1972). Effects of topical chemoprophylaxis on transferable antibiotic resistance in burns. *Lancet*, **1**, 109

23 Casewell, M. W. (1979). Transfer of antibiotic resistance between *Klebsiella, E. coli, Proteus mirabilis,* and *Citrobacter* species in the urinary tract of a patient. (In preparation)

24 Editorial. (1973). Chloramphenicol resistance in typhoid. *Lancet*, **2**, 1008

25 Schiffer, M. S., MacLowry, J., Schneerson, R. and Robbins, J. B. (1974). Clinical, bacteriological and immunological characterisation of ampicillin-resistant *Haemophilus influenzae* type B. *Lancet*, **2**, 257

26 Percival, A., Rowlands, J., Corkill, J. E., Alergant, C. D., Arya, O. A., Rees, E. and

Annels, E. H. (1976). Penicillinase-producing gonococci in Liverpool. *Lancet*, **2**, 1379

27 Appelbaum, P. C., Bhamjee, A., Scragg, J. N., Hallett, A. J., Bowen, A. J. and Cooper, R. C. (1977). Streptococcus pneumoniae resistant to penicillin and chloramphenicol. *Lancet*, **2**, 995

28 Wood, H. F., Feinstein, A. R., Taranta, A., Epstein, J. A. and Simpson, R. (1964). Rheumatic fever in children and adolescents. A long-term epidemiologic study of subsequent prophylaxis, streptococcal infections, and clinical sequelae. III. Comparative effectiveness of three prophylaxis regimens in preventing streptococcal infections and rheumatic recurrences. *Ann. Intern. Med.*, **60** (Suppl. 5), 31

29 Editorial. (1967). Rheumatic heart disease. *Lancet*, **1**, 29

30 Standing Medical Advisory Committee for the Central Health Services and the Minister of Health. (1965). *Prevention of Initial Attacks and Recurrences of Rheumatic Fever.* (Ministry of Health)

31 Epidemiology Unit No. 22. (1945). Sulfadiazine resistant strains of beta-haemolytic streptococci. *J. Am. Med. Assoc.*, **129**, 921

32 Phillips, I., Warren, C., Harrison, J. M., Sharples, P., Ball, L. C. and Parker, M. T. (1976). Antibiotic susceptibilities of streptococci from the mouth and blood of patients treated with penicillin or lincomycin and clindamycin. *J. Med. Microbiol.*, **9**, 393

33 Shanson, D. C., Cannon, P. and Wilks, M. (1978). Amoxycillin compared with penicillin V for the prophylaxis of dental bacteraemia. *J. Antimicrob. Chemother.*, **4**, 431

34 Pelletier, L. L., Durack, D. T. and Petersdorf, R. G. (1975). Chemotherapy of experimental streptococcal endocarditis. IV. Further observations on prophylaxis. *J. Clin. Invest.*, **56**, 319

35 Petersdorf, R. G. (1978). Antimicrobial prophylaxis of bacterial endocarditis. Prudent caution or bacterial overkill? *Am. J. Med.*, **65**, 220

36 Phillips, I. and Eykyn, S. (1973). Bacterial endocarditis following cardiac surgery. In A. M. Geddes and J. D. Williams (eds.) *Current Antibiotic Therapy*, pp. 113–123. (Edinburgh and London: Churchill Livingstone)

37 Newsom, S. W. B. (1978). Antibiotic prophylaxis for open-heart surgery. *J. Antimicrob. Chemother.*, **4**, 389

38 Leading article. ((1969). Post-operative gas gangrene. *Brit. Med. J.*, **3**, 665

39 Parker, M. T. (1969). Postoperative clostridial infections in Britain. *Brit. Med. J.*, **3**, 671

40 Artenstein, M. S. Lamson, T. H. and Evans, J. R. (1967). Attempted prophylaxis against meningococcal infection using intramuscular penicillin. *Milit. Med.*, **132**, 1009

41 News and Notes (1976). Epidemiology. Meningococcal meningitis in England and Wales. *Brit. Med. J.*, **2**, 430

42 Beam, W. E., Newberg, N. R., Devine, L. F., Pierce, W. E. and Davies, J. A. (1971. The effect of rifampicin on the nasopharyngeal carriage of *Neisseria meningitidis* in a military population. *J. Infect. Dis.*, **124**, 39

43 Guttler, R. B. and Beaty, H. N. (1972). Minocycline in the chemoprophylaxis of meningococcal disease. *Antimicrob. Agents Chemother.*, **1**, 397

44 Williams, D. N., Laughlin, L. W. and Lee, Y. (1974). Minocycline: possible vestibular side-effects. *Lancet*, **2**, 744

45 Abbott, J. D., Simmons, L. E., Ironside, A. G., Mandal, B. K., Fraser Williams, R., Brennand, J., Mann, N. M. and Simon, S. (1974). Diphtheria in the Manchester area 1967–1971. *Lancet*, **2**, 1558

46 McCloskey, R. V., Eller, J. J., Green, M., Mauney, C. U. and Richards, S. E. M. (1971). The 1970 epidemic of diphtheria in San Antonio. *Ann. Intern. Med.*, **75**, 495

47 Evans, A. J. (1975). The modern treatment of burns. *Br. J. Hosp. Med.*, **13**, 287

48 Lowbury, E. J. L., Jackson, D. M., Lilly, H. A., Bull, J. P., Cason, J. S., Davies, J. W. L. and Ford, P. M. (1971). Alternative forms of local treatment for burns. *Lancet*, **2**, 1105

49 Editorial (1978). Infection after hip replacement. *Lancet*, **1**, 482

50 Charnley, J. and Eftekhar, N. (1969). Postoperative infection in total prosthetic replacement arthoplasty of the hip-joint. *Br. J. Surg.*, **56**, 641

51 Fitzgerald, R. H., Peterson, L. F. A., Washington, J. A., Van Scoy, R. E. and Coventry, M. B. (1973). Bacterial colonization of wounds and sepsis in total hip arthoplasty. *J. Bone Joint Surg.*, **55A**, 1242

52 Ericson, C., Lidgren, L. and Lindberg, L. (1973). Cloxacillin in the prophylaxis of postoperative infections of the hip. *J. Bone Joint Surg.*, **55A**, 808

53 Unsworth, P. F., Heatley, F. W. and Phillips, I. (1978). Flucloxacillin in bone. *J. Clin. Path.*, **31**, 705

54 Hughes, S. P. F., Benson, M. K. D., Dash, C. H. and Field, C. A. (1975). Cephaloridine penetration into bone and synovial capsule of patients undergoing hip joint replacement. *J. Antimicrob. Chemother.*, **1** (Suppl.), 41

55 Hughes, S. P. F., Want, S., Darrell, J. H., Dash, C. H. and Kennedy, M. R. K. (1978). The penetration of cefuroxime into bone. In *The Early Evaluation of Cefuroxime*, Proceedings of Symposium, 1977, p. 83. (Greenford, Middlesex: Glaxo Laboratories Ltd.)

56 Moore, B. (1977). Antibiotics in cement. *J. Bone Joint Surg.*, **59B**, 139

57 Tabaqchali, S. (1974). Ecology and metabolic activity of non-sporing anaerobes. In I. Phillips and M. Sussman (eds.) *Infection with Non-sporing Anaerobic Bacteria*, pp. 59–90. (Edinburgh, London and New York: Churchill Livingstone)

58 Leigh, D. A. (1974). Clinical importance of infections due to *Bacteroides fragilis* and role of antibiotic therapy. *Brit. Med. J.*, **1**, 225

59 French, J. cited by Williams, J. A. (1973). Prophylactic use of antibiotics in surgery. In A. M. Geddes and J. D. Williams (eds.). *Current Antibiotic Therapy*, pp. 142–145. (Edinburgh and London: Churchill Livingstone)

60 Editorial. (1970). The colon and the surgeon. *Lancet*, **1**, 509

61 Polk, H. C. and Lopez-Mayor, J. F. (1969). Postoperative wound infection: a prospective study of determinant factors and prevention. *Surgery*, **66**, 97

62 Stokes, E. J., Waterworth, P. M., Franks, V., Watson, B. and Clark, C. G. (1974). Short term routine prophylaxis in surgery. *Brit. J. Surg.*, **61**, 739

63 Willis, A. T., Ferguson, I. R., Jones, P. H., Phillips, K. D., Tearle, P. V., Berry, R. B., Fiddian, R. V., Graham, D. F., Harland, D. H. C., Innes, D. B., Mee, W. M., Rothwell-Jackson, R. L., Sutch, I., Kilbey, C. and Edwards, D. (1976). Metronidazole in prevention and treatment of bacteroides infections after appendicectomy. *Brit. Med. J.*, **1**, 318

64 Willis, A. T., Ferguson, I. R., Jones, P. H., Phillips, K. D., Tearle, P. V., Fiddian, R. V., Graham, D. F., Harland, D. H. C., Hughes, D. F. R., Knight, D., Mee, W. M., Pashby, N., Rothwell-Jackson, R. L., Sachdeva, A. K., Sutch, I., Kilbey, C. and Edwards, D. (1977). Metronidazole in prevention and treatment of bacteroides infections in elective colonic surgery. *Brit. Med. J.*, **1**, 607

65 Report of a Study Group. (1975). An evaluation of metronidazole in the prophylaxis and treatment of anaerobic sepsis in surgical patients. *J. Antimicrob. Chemother.*, **1**, 393

66   Kappas, A., Shinagawa, N., Arabi, Y., Thompson, H., Burdon, D. W., Dimock, F., George, R. H., Alexander-Williams, J. and Keighley, M. R. B. (1978). Diagnosis of pseudomembranous colitis. *Brit. Med. J.*, **1**, 675

67   Clark, C. E., Thompson, H., McLeish, A. R., Powis, S. J. A., Dorricott, N. J. and Alexander-Williams, J. (1976). Pseudomembranous colitis following prophylactic antibiotics in bowel surgery. *J. Antimicrob. Chemother.*, **2**, 167

68   Feathers, R. S., Lewis, A. A. M., Sagor, G. R., Amirak, I. D. and Noone, P. (1977). Prophylactic systemic antibiotics in colorectal surgery. *Lancet*, **1**, 4

69   Griffiths, D. A., Shorey, B. A., Simpson, R. A., Speller, D. C. E. and Williams, N. B. (1976). Single-dose peroperative antibiotic prophylaxis in gastro-intestinal surgery. *Lancet*, **2**, 325

70   Galland, R. B., Saunders, J. H., Mosley, J. G. and Darrell, J. H. (1977). Prevention of wound infection in abdominal operations by peroperative antibiotics or povidone-iodine. A controlled trial. *Lancet*, **2**, 1043

71   Casewell, M. W. and Eykyn, S. (1978). (Unpublished)

72   Bailey, R. R., Roberts, A. P., Gower, P. E. and de Wardener, H. E. (1971). Prevention of urinary-tract infection with low-dose nitrofurantoin. *Lancet*, **2**, 1112

73   Harding, G. K. M. and Ronald, A. R. (1974). A controlled study of antimicrobial prophylaxis of recurrent urinary infections in women. *New Engl. J. Med.*, **291**, 597

74   Smellie, J. M., Grüneberg, R. N., Leakey, A. and Atkin, W. S. (1976). Long-term low-dose co-trimoxazole in prophylaxis of childhood urinary tract infections: Clinical aspects. *Brit. Med. J.*, **2**, 203

75   Leading Article. (1974). Chemoprophylaxis against tuberculosis. *Brit. Med. J.*, **4**, 63

76   World Health Organisation (1976). Information on Malaria Risk for International Travellers. *Weekly Epidemiological Record*, **51**, 181

77   U.S. Department of Health, Education, and Welfare. Public Health Service. Center for Disease Control. *Health Information for International Travel 1978.* (HEW Publication No. (CDC) 78–8280)

78   Editorial. (1978). Infection prevention in acute leukaemia. *Lancet*, **2**, 768

79   Gurwith, M. (1978). Prevention of infection in leukaemia, *J. Antimicrob. Chemother*, **4**, 302

80   Storring, R. A., Jameson, B., McElwain, T. J., Wiltshaw, E., Spiers, A. S. D. and Gaya, H. (1977). Oral non-absorbed antibiotics prevent infection in acute non-lymphoblastic leukaemia. *Lancet*, **2**, 837

81   Gurwith, M. J., Brunton, J. L., Lank, B. A., Harding, G. K. M., Ronald, A. (1977). Prophylactic trimethoprim/sulphamethoxazole (TMP/SMZ) in granulocytopenic patients. *Proc. XVIII Intersci. Conf. Antimicrob. Agents Chemother.*, abstr. 409. (New York)

82   Hughes, D. (1976). Chemoprophylaxis in chronic bronchitis. *J. Antimicrob. Chemother*, **2**, 320

3

The cephalosporin group of antibiotics

Rosamund J. Williams and J. D. Williams

HISTORICAL INTRODUCTION

The remarkable growth in the development of the cephalosporin group of antibiotics stems from the isolation of cephalosporin C in 1955[1]. The recognition of the active agents, however, preceded this by some years. In 1945, Brotzu, at that time Rector in the Sicilian University of Cagliari, noted that the seawater near a sewage outlet in that town appeared to be self-purifying and proposed that this might be due in part to bacterial antagonism. Brotzu examined the microbial flora of the seawater and isolated a fungus which he concluded to be similar to *Cephalosporium acremonium*. This fungus appeared to have an inhibitory effect on certain bacteria *in vitro* and Brotzu used the crude products of its growth with some success for treating typhoid fever and brucellosis. In 1948 he published his findings in a journal that he founded for the purpose since no other learned journal would accept the work[2]. He also sent a culture of his fungus to Oxford in England.

In 1949 two groups of workers[3 4] in England started to examine the culture fluids from Brotzu's fungus and recognised two active substances; cephalosporin P and cephalosporin N. In 1952, cephalosporin N was shown to be a new type of penicillin and a purified sample yielded penicillamine on acid hydrolysis[5]. It was later renamed penicillin N. Cephalosporin P was found to have a steroid structure similar to fusidic acid[6]. The next year a second hydrophilic antibiotic was discovered in the metabolic products of the *Cephalosporium* sp. This was named cephalosporin C. Early studies showed that cephalosporin C could be separated from impure penicillin N but it was present in such small amounts in the culture fluids from the Sardinian *Cephalosporium* sp.

that it could not be detected by antibacterial assay and had only been discovered because it was concentrated during the purification of penicillin N.

By 1955 studies on the antibacterial activity of cephalosporin C were under way. It was shown to have a wide range of activity and to be equally effective against strains of penicillin-resistant and penicillin-sensitive staphylococci. It was innocuous to mice when given intravenously in large doses, and it would protect them against experimental streptococcal infection when the antibiotic was administered subcutaneously[7]. By 1957, the potential importance of cephalosporin C, especially its resistance to penicillinase, had been recognised. In 1959 the structure of cephalosporin C was proposed and later confirmed by X-ray crystallography, and small amounts of 7-aminocephalosporanic acid were isolated in a relatively pure form (Figure 1). The N-phenylacetyl derivative was shown to be much more active than cephalosporin C itself against penicillinase-producing strains of *Staphylococcus aureus*[8]. In 1960, a chemical procedure was discovered by Lilly Research

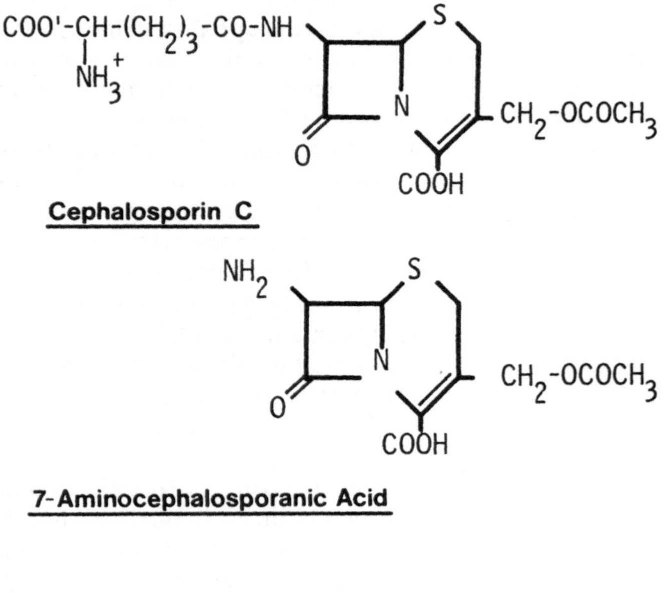

Cephalosporin C

7-Aminocephalosporanic Acid

Figure 1

Laboratories that produced 7-aminocephalosporanic acid in much higher yields and from then on chemical manipulations were undertaken to improve the performance of the cephalosporins. So the first stages of the discovery and isolation of cephalosporins were slow, but since then the field of cephalosporin antibiotics has blossomed with much greater rapidity.

The cephalosporin nucleus contains several positions where chemical modification can be made (Figure 2) and many thousands of cephalosporin compounds have been produced by various pharmaceutical companies around the world.

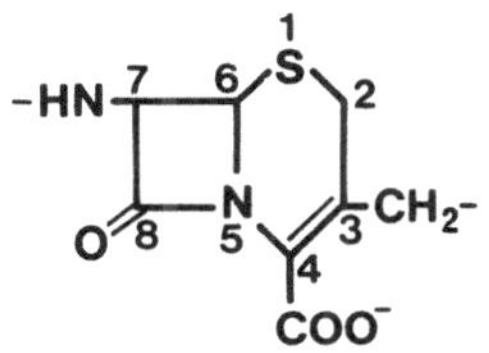

Figure 2 Numbered positions on the cephalosporin nucleus where chemical modification can be made

Most of the early modification efforts were directed at the 7-acyl group because it was soon realised that this substituent largely determined the kind and amount of antibacterial activity possessed by an analogue. Substitution at the 3 position affected mainly pharmacokinetic properties. However there is considerable interaction between the two groups and it is often impossible to predict the properties of a new analogue.

Thus early in cephalosporin research, substitution was usually at the 7 position leaving the 3-acetoxy group in place. Later the effects of changes at the 3 position were explored. This has lead to the evolution of several main groups of cephalosporins (Figure 3).

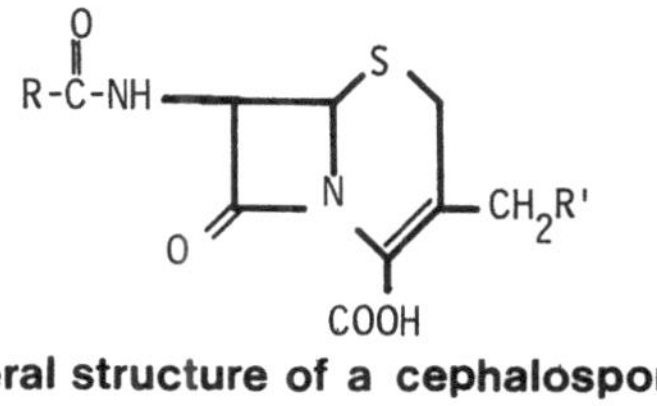

General structure of a cephalosporin

Figure 3   Chemical classification of cephalosporins

1. 3-acetoxymethyl cephalosporins

CEPHALOTHIN

CEPHAPIRIN

CEPHACETRILE

2. Ester replaced in position 3

CEPHALORIDINE

CEFAZOLIN

3. Orally-absorbed cephalosporins

CEPHALEXIN

CEPHRADINE

CEFACLOR

4. βeta-lactamase resistant cephalosporins

CEFAMANDOLE

CEFUROXIME

CEFOTAXIME

5. Cephamycins

CEFOXITIN

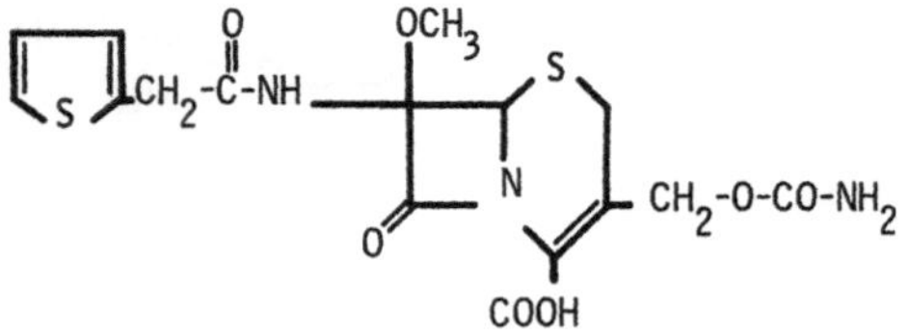

6. Unclassified

CEFSULODIN

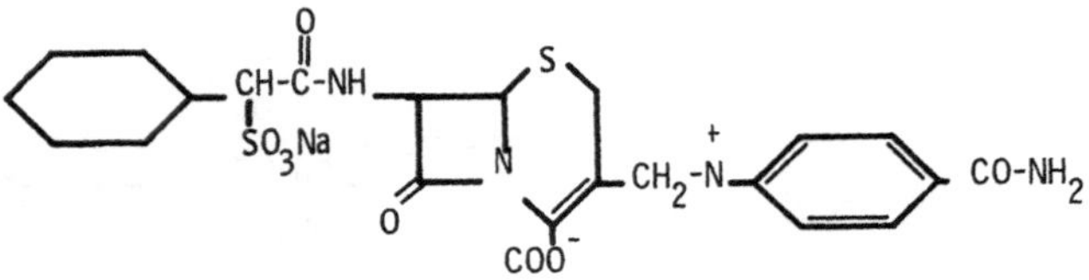

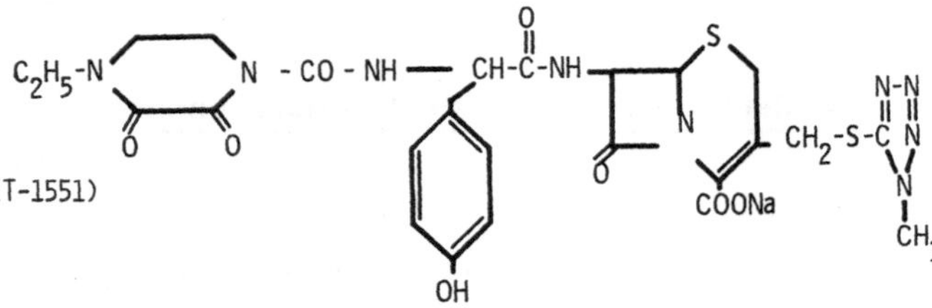

CEFOPERAZONE (T-1551)

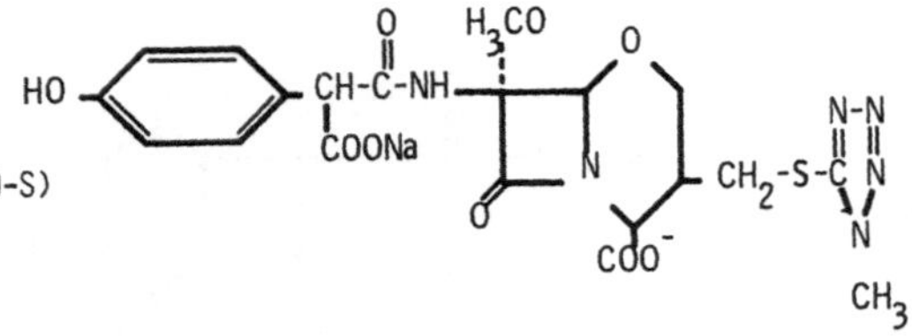

LY 127935 (6059-S)

Firstly, the 3-acetoxymethyl cephalosporins, of which cephalothin was the first to be made available for clinical use, followed later by cephapirin and cephacetrile. However, all such cephalosporins with the acetoxy group in the 3 position were found to be unstable in the body and were converted by esterases to the corresponding deacetyl component which has low antibacterial activity. This problem was overcome in the second group of cephalosporins by replacing the ester group at position 3. This led in 1964 to the introduction of cephaloridine and some time later, cefazolin.

It was found that oral absorption of cephalosporins was due to both the a-amino group in the 7-acyl substituent and to the small uncharged group in position 3. The first of the orally-absorbable cephalosporins, cephalexin, was introduced in 1969. Later followed cephradine, and in 1978, cefaclor.

The greatest challenge to cephalosporin development has really arisen in the need to devise cephalosporins that are resistant to the action of β-lactamases. Because there is such a variety of types of β-lactamases it has proved difficult to modify the β-lactam structure in such a way as to make it insensitive to all enzymes while retaining antibacterial efficacy. The ring system of cephalosporins greatly influences hydrolysis. It is the nature of the substituent at the 7-acyl position which seems to have the primary influence on the susceptibility of the molecule to β-lactamase. The presence of $-CH_2-$ next to the amide link is almost always accompanied by sensitivity to the β-lactamases of Gram-negative organisms but this decreases as steric hindrance is introduced. The steric effects are greater on Gram-negative β-lactamases than on those from Gram-positive organisms. Once the 7-acyl group has introduced a degree of resistance, alteration at the 3 position does not alter this resistance and may enhance it. The first of the β-lactamase resistant cephalosporins to be brought into clinical use was cefamandole, followed by cefuroxime. Both these cephalosporins have large groupings substituted at the 7-acyl position (see Figure 3).

In the search for β-lactamase-stable cephalosporins a group of compounds similar but not the same as cephalosporins has emerged; the cephamycins. The first of these compounds to be introduced clinically is cefoxitin. Cefoxitin is a naturally occurring substance produced by *Streptomyces lactamdurans*. It is structurally similar to cephalothin but has an additional 7-a-methoxy group which renders it resistant to hydrolysis by most β-lactamases of Gram-negative and Gram-positive bacteria.

A new development has been the production of several cephalosporins showing antibacterial activity against *Pseudomonas aeruginosa*. The chemical relationships of these compounds are unclear at present and therefore we have put them in an unclassified group. All three shown in Figure 3 have a second substituent on the 7β-carbon atom and one, LY 127935 (6059-S), contains O substituted for S in the cephalosporin nucleus.

MODE OF ACTION

Penicillins and cephalosporins interfere with the synthesis of the mucopeptide (peptidoglycan) component of the bacterial cell wall. The synthesis of bacterial cell walls takes place in three distinct stages at three different sites in the cell[9]. It is the third stage, which occurs outside the cell membrane, which is specifically inhibited by penicillins and cephalosporins. At this stage the linear peptidoglycan strands are cross-linked by a transpeptidation step in which a peptide bridge is formed between two adjacent strands, with the elimination of D-alanine. It is postulated that β-lactam might be a structural analogue of the D-*alanyl*-D-alanine end of the peptide chain. If the transpeptidase formed an acyl intermediate with the end of the pentapeptide, eliminating D-alanine, it could also react with penicillin forming a penicilloyl intermediate and thus become inactivated[10].

Gram-negative bacilli have in addition a carboxypeptidase enzyme involved in terminal peptidoglycan synthesis. This is also inhibited by penicillins and cephalosporins but the reaction is reversible[11]. The concentration of penicillin required to inhibit carboxypeptidase is considerably less than that required to inhibit growth of the organism, whereas concentrations required to inhibit transpeptidase are of the same order as those which prevent bacterial growth. It therefore seems likely that the primary effect of β-lactam antibiotics is the inhibition of the transpeptidase. Bacterial cells must be actively dividing before inhibitors of cell wall synthesis can be effective.

Most penicillins and cephalosporins investigated to date appear to have similar modes of action but there are considerable differences in the killing rates. There are probably several types of peptidoglycan synthesis in bacterial cells and this may in part account for the variability in sensitivity of bacteria to β-lactam antibiotics, and for the variety of effects that β-lactam antibiotics appear to have on cells. With the Gram-negative bacilli, β-lactam antibiotics exert effects on the cell morphology which are concentration dependent. Low antibiotic concentrations tend to lead to the formation of filamentous cells, often many times the length of the normal bacilli. High concentrations result in cell elongation, spheroplast formation and lysis[12] [13].

At a stage in peptidoglycan synthesis it is necessary for lytic enzymes to open a part of the cell wall and permit insertion of a new piece of peptidoglycan. In the presence of a β-lactam antibiotic the lytic enzymes will continue to function normally although cell wall synthesis is inhibited. This results in an increase in the permeability of the cell, leading eventually to lysis.

Blumberg and Strominger[14] suggested that filament formation and rupture of the swollen regions of such cells results from the inhibition of a transpeptidase involved in cross-wall formation and this occurs at the minimum lethal concentration of antibiotic. In contrast, rapid lysis in the absence of filament formation may be due to inhibition of a different transpeptidase which is also involved in the division process. It is postulated that with some β-lactams, e.g. amoxycillin and cephaloridine, the second enzyme is inhibited at concentrations only slightly greater than those that inhibit the first. This results in the rapid onset of lysis without prior filament formation. In contrast, with cephalexin the second enzyme is only inhibited at antibiotic concentrations much greater than those that inhibit septation. So the tendency is for cells to form filaments and only lyse at high cephalexin concentrations.

Spratt[13] reported that the effects of β-lactam antibiotics on the morphology of *Escherichia coli* were due to their interactions with essential penicillin binding proteins with distinct roles. For various binding sites on the cell membrane the binding constant varies from one cephalosporin to another. Mutation in the gene which specifies the nature of the binding site, i.e. the target, will result in resistance to the antibiotic but if the β-lactam attacks more than one target, then total resistance would require a coordinated set of mutations.

The variation in morphological response to different β-lactams may have some clinical significance. Rolinson and colleagues[15] showed that filamentous forms of *E. coli* were capable of resuming cell division very rapidly if the antibiotic was removed before the cells lyse. Characteristically, β-lactam antibiotics are eliminated rapidly from the body and thus the period of time for which they are present in concentrations sufficient to lyse the cells at the site of infection may be short. Thus cells that develop filamentous forms in response to the antibiotic could survive.

MECHANISMS OF RESISTANCE TO CEPHALOSPORINS

The resistance of bacteria to the cephalosporins depends on two major factors and the interactions between them:

the existence of a permeability barrier to the penetration of the antibiotic into the site of peptidoglycan synthesis;
the production of enzymes that destroy the antibiotic.

The permeability barrier
The structures of the outer envelopes of Gram-positive and Gram-

GRAM-NEGATIVE CELL WALL

β-lactam antibiotic

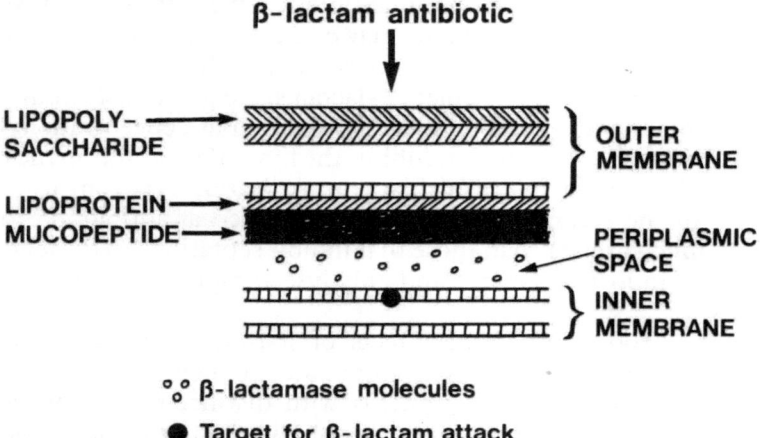

LIPOPOLY-SACCHARIDE

LIPOPROTEIN

MUCOPEPTIDE

OUTER MEMBRANE

PERIPLASMIC SPACE

INNER MEMBRANE

°₀° β-lactamase molecules

● Target for β-lactam attack

GRAM-POSITIVE CELL WALL

β-lactam antibiotic

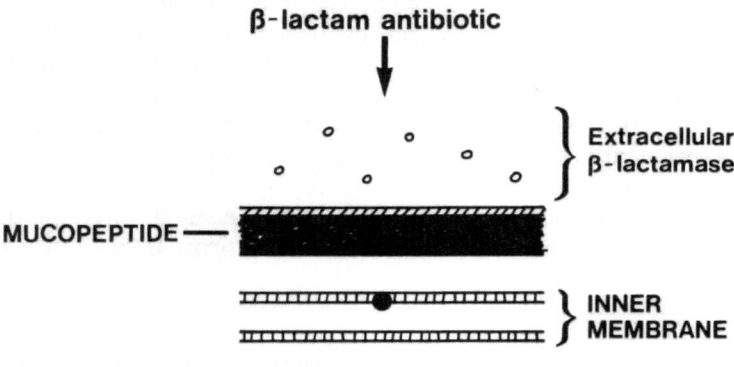

MUCOPEPTIDE

Extracellular β-lactamase

INNER MEMBRANE

● Target for β-lactam attack

Figure 4

negative cells are considerably different and are shown diagrammatically in Figure 4. Many Gram-positive organisms have relatively simple cell walls lying outside the cell membrane. The major and constant component of the cell wall is mucopeptide or peptidoglycan which forms at least 50% of the wall mass. Other wall components are more variable. Thus, the target for cephalosporin attack, the peptidoglycan, is superficially placed on the cell and relatively easily accessible; therefore the permeability barrier is of little consequence in the resistance of Gram-positive organisms to cephalosporins.

The outer layers of Gram-negative cells comprise an envelope of lipoprotein attached to the underlying peptidoglycan, an outer membrane with a typical lipid bi-layer structure and, closely associated with the outer face of this membrane, is the lipopolysaccharide which bears the oligosaccharide chains which determine the antigenic specificity of Gram-negative organisms. The most important determinants of permeability to drugs in Gram-negative organisms appear to be the outer membrane and the lipopolysaccharide. This permeability barrier has the effect of restricting the rate at which the cephalosporin can reach its target sites. The nature of the barrier may be species specific. For example, strains of *Ps. aeruginosa* have a barrier which excludes penicillins and cephalosporins, whereas in some strains of *E. coli* the barrier excludes penicillin but not cephaloridine. Strains of *Haemophilus influenzae* do not exclude either penicillins or cephalosporins.

Beta-lactamases

There are several ways in which β-lactam antibiotics can be inactivated by enzymes (Figure 5) but the only one of importance involves the opening of the β-lactam ring; a hydrolysis reaction catalysed by β-lactamases. These enzymes include both penicillinases and cephalosporinases. With penicillins such hydrolysis yields penicilloic acid, but

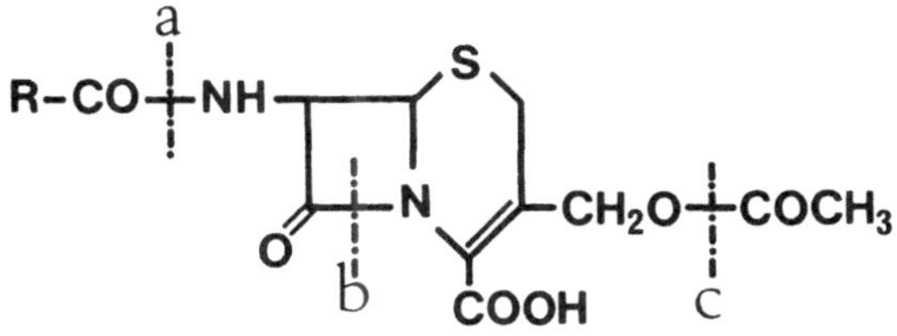

a   = amidase

b   = beta-lactamase

c   = esterase

Figure 5 Sites of enzymatic cleavage in cephalosporins

with cephalosporins the intermediate cephalosporic acid is unstable and undergoes rapid decomposition to yield products, the nature of which depends on the relative strengths of the acidic and basic groups of the cephalosporin molecule (Figure 6). To date no β-lactamase has been

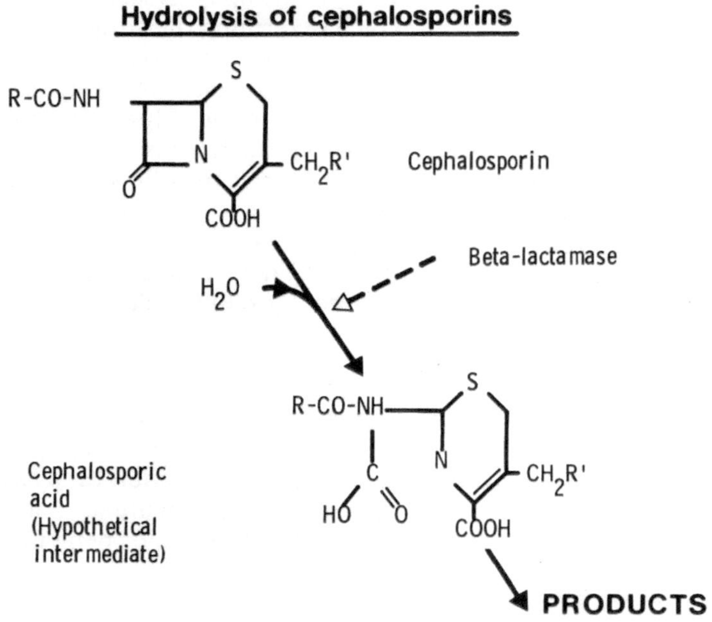

Hydrolysis of cephalosporins

R-CO-NH

Cephalosporin

H₂O

Beta-lactamase

R-CO-NH

Cephalosporic
acid
(Hypothetical
intermediate)

PRODUCTS

Figure 6 Hydrolysis of cephalosporins

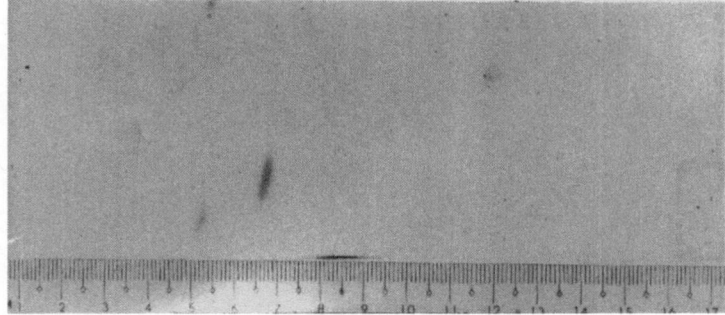

Figure 7 Isoelectric focussing of β-lactamases produced by subspecies of *Bacteroides fragilis*. 1, ss. *fragilis* pH 4.9. 2, *distasonis* pH 5.1. 3, ss. *thetaiotaomicron* pH 4.5. 4, ss. *vulgatus* pH 4.6. 5, ss. *ovatus* pH 6.7

Table 1 Hydrolysis by *B. fragilis* subsp β-lactamases of 7 cephalosporins, and cefoxitin

	ss. *fragilis*			ss. *ovatus*	ss. *vulgatus*	ss. *theta iotaomicron*	ss. *diastonis*
	a	b	c				
Cephaloridine	0.016 (100)	0.14 (100)	0.13 (100)	0.1 (100)	0.14 (100)	0.02 (100)	0.2 (100)
Cephalothin	0.015 (94)	0.13 (98)	0.05 (36)	0.07 (70)	0.03 (21)	0.03 (140)	0.33 (122)
Cefazolin	0.02 (128)	0.11 (76)	0.03 (28)	0.032 (32)	0.04 (28)	0.04 (180)	0.11 (56)
Cephamandole	0.01 (58)	0.009 (64)	0.03 (23)	0.04 (40)	–	–	0.07 (26)
Cephalexin	0.005 (29)	0.04 (28)	0.024 (18)	0.001 (10)	0.03 (20)	–	0.07 (26)
Cephradine	0.004 (22)	0.04 (38)	0.023 (15)	0.002 (15)	0.035 (25)	–	0.05 (25)
Cefuroxime	0.012 (75)	0.03 (18)	–	0.05 (50)	–	–	0.04 (22)
Cefoxitin	0 (0)	0 (0)	0 (0)	0 (0)	0 (0)	–	0 (0)

Specific activity expressed in μmol hydrolysed per min per mg protein (and relative % hydrolysis compared to cephaloridine)
– = Not tested

described which is exclusively a penicillinase or a cephalosporinase. A β-lactamase which has high activity against penicillins also shows low activity against cephalosporins and vice versa.

It is probable that all bacteria produce at least one chromosomally-mediated β-lactamase and it is presumed that these enzymes play a part in the cell's normal physiology. The chromosomally-mediated β-lactamases are specific for the genus, species and sub-species of bacteria[16], and β-lactamases produced by different bacterial species have widely varying substrate specificities (Table 1). The great majority of chromosomally-mediated β-lactamases are primarily cephalosporinases and these enzymes usually hydrolyse susceptible cephalosporins 5–10 times as rapidly as they hydrolyse benzyl penicillin. Several bacterial strains constitutively produce exceptionally high levels of β-lactamase, whereas others produce very low levels, e.g. *Bordetella bronchiseptica*, *Haemophilus influenzae* and *Neisseria gonorrhoeae*. In some genera production of the enzyme is inducible by β-lactam substrates[17], or by β-lactamase inhibitors[18], or sometimes by substances which fall into neither of these two groups[19].

The genetic coding for β-lactamase production may also be plasmid-borne. There appear to be thousands of such plasmids but they seem to code for only a few different β-lactamases[16]. The introduction of such a plasmid into a cell increases β-lactamase production to a far higher level than that produced by chromosomally-mediated enzymes. Thus, plasmid-mediated β-lactamases of identical characteristics are found in many bacterial species (Figure 7).

In Gram-positive organisms, resistance to β-lactam antibiotics is almost entirely due to production of relatively large amounts of β-lactamases with high affinity for the β-lactam substrates concerned. These enzymes are extracellular and are liberated into the surrounding medium, destroying the antibiotic before it reaches the cell surface. Under these circumstances the enzyme can be greatly diluted, thus the need for a high level of enzyme production. A single cell alone is defenceless and the resistance of the population depends on the production of β-lactamase by the mass of bacteria.

So far, no cephalosporin has been found to be as sensitive to staphylococcal β-lactamase as is benzyl penicillin. Cephalothin shows almost total resistance to staphylococcal β-lactamase but cephaloridine is rather less resistant. The orally-absorbed cephalosporins, cephaloglycin and cephalexin, also show a high degree of stability to the staphylococcal enzymes and cefazolin and cephapirin are almost completely unaffected.

The β-lactamases of Gram-negative bacteria have been reviewed in detail[20][21]. Gram-negative β-lactamases are generally produced constitutively in very much smaller amounts than are found in Gram-positive organisms. Under physiological conditions the enzymes are cell-bound and are not released into the surrounding medium. These enzymes have low substrate affinities compared with the β-lactamases produced by Gram-positive organisms. Certain genera, e.g. *Enterobacter, Citrobacter,* some *Proteus* sp. and *Providencia,* have inducible β-lactamases and thus produce considerable amounts of enzyme. Resistance to cephalosporins due to enzyme production in Gram-negative organisms depends largely on the level of enzyme production and this may be altered by induction, mutation, or by acquisition of a specific R-plasmid coding for β-lactamase production.

The *Enterobacteriaceae* produce such a plethora of β-lactamases that various attempts have been made to classify them into groups. Sykes and Matthew[20] grouped β-lactamases firstly according to whether they were normally mediated chromosomally or by transmissible R-plasmids, and secondly by their substrate profile. The stability of various cephalosporins to one enzyme or the activity of various enzymes on one cephalosporin can be studied by monitoring the changes in ultra-violet absorption spectra of cephalosporins following β-lactamase hydrolysis (Table 2). Thus cephalosporins can be classified according to their sensitivity to β-lactamases. The recent introduction of β-lactamase-stable cephalosporins has helped to overcome the problem of resistance to cephalosporins as a result of destruction by β-lactamase. Cefuroxime and cefoxitin are not inactivated by the majority of β-lactamases and consequently show antibacterial activity against β-lactamase-producing *Enterobacteriaceae*.

Table 2 Hydrolysis of cephalosporins by β-lactamases of Gram-negative bacilli

	Enzymes					
Cephalosporin	R_{TEM}	RPl	Kl	P99	Bact.	Proteus M
Cephaloridine	100	100	100	100	100	100
Cephalothin	14	12	34	29	175	15
Cefazolin	7	9	61	15	22	15
Cefamandole	107	114	201	0	?	115
Cephalexin	0	0	0	29	?	0
Cephradine	0	0	0	16	0	0
Cefotaxime	0	0	0.2	0	0	0
Cefuroxime	0	0	0.6	0	0	0
Cefoxitin	0	0	0	0	0	0

Relative % hydrolysis compared to cephaloridine
(Leung and Williams; unpublished data)

Crypticity
In the majority of instances the permeability barrier and the production of β-lactamase work together to make a cell resistant to a cephalosporin. The measurement of crypticity relies on the fact that β-lactamases of Gram-negative bacteria are cell-bound enzymes located behind a permeability barrier, probably in the periplasmic space (Figure 4). Under normal conditions β-lactamase cannot pass out of the cell and therefore before any interaction between enzyme and substrate can take place the antibiotic molecule must penetrate the permeability barrier. If this is achieved, then the fate of the cell rests with the β-lactamase; concentration of enzyme, affinity for its substrate, and rate of substrate hydrolysis all play an important role.

Crypticity can be expressed as:

$$\text{Crypticity} = \frac{\text{specific enzymic activity of broken cells}}{\text{specific enzymic activity of whole cells}}$$

When measured in this way, crypticity is a function of the barrier and of the kinetics of the enzyme concerned. A high crypticity value indicates the presence of a barrier to the antibiotic under test, although a low crypticity value does not exclude this possibility[20].

ANTIBACTERIAL ACTIVITY

Assessment of antibacterial activity of cephalosporins
There are many methods of assessing the antibacterial activity of antibiotics. The aim of *in vitro* susceptibility testing is to predict as accurately as possible the *in vivo* activity of an agent. Cephalosporins provide peculiar difficulties in assessment because of their complex mode of action and because of the various mechanisms of resistance to them. Reference has been made in an earlier section to the three components of cephalosporin activity – the penetration of the outer layers of the bacterial cell; the affinity for, and ability to interfere with, the target site inside the periplasmic space; and the stability of the cephalosporin to chromosomally- and plasmid-mediated β-lactamases. It is difficult to determine which laboratory susceptibility tests most accurately reflect the combined effect of these three factors, and some such difficulties are shown in Table 3. *In vitro*, if there is a readily penetrable barrier, the antibiotic may diffuse so rapidly into the cell that the latter is killed before any β-lactamase present has had the opportunity to act.

But *in vivo* the antibiotic may be delivered to the cells more slowly than in a laboratory experiment, and the β-lactamase may be able to inactivate the antibiotic. For example, ampicillin may inhibit penicillinase-producing *H. influenzae in vitro* at low concentrations when small inocula are tested because there is little barrier to penetration[22]. However, when large inocula are tested, as would be present *in vivo* for example in the meninges, the organisms are not responsive to ampicillin.

The effect of the β-lactamase contribution to the outcome of cephalosporin–organism interaction is difficult to assess and varies considerably with the test conditions. In Table 3, where small inocula were tested, it appears that the presence of a TEM β-lactamase, which is capable of hydrolysing many cephalosporins, does not produce a major change in MIC or in zone size in disc diffusion tests.

In attempting to review the large volume of information on the antibacterial activity of cephalosporins, we have been unable to provide data on antibacterial activity which is closely related to *in vivo* response in man. Most studies confine themselves to MICs for a variety of bacteria and it is from such data that we must predict 'resistance' or

Table 3 Relationship of hydrolysis by β-lactamase, possession of a permeability barrier and MIC to outcome of treatment*

Antibiotic	Strain	β-lactamase hydrolysis	Barrier	MIC (μg/ml)	Zone size	Clinical response
Ampicillin	E. coli	−	+	1–2	Large	Yes
	E. coli	+	+	128	None	No
	H. influenzae	−	−	0.25	Large	Yes
	H. influenzae	+	−	2	Slight reduction	No
Cephaloridine	E. coli	−	−	1–2	Large	Yes
	E. coli	+	−	4–8	Slight reduction	No
	H. influenzae	−	+	4–8	Small	No
	H. influenzae	+	+	8–16	Small	No
	B. fragilis	−	−	0.5	Large	Yes
	B. fragilis	−	+	16	Moderate	No
	B. fragilis	+	+	128	None	No

* from Williams, J. D. (1978). The correlation of *in vitro* susceptibility tests with *in vivo* results of antibiotic treatment. *Scand. J. Infect. Dis.* (Suppl.), **13**, 64

'susceptibility' of organisms *in vivo*. This may be clear, but often the MICs for members of a bacterial species extend over a wide range. To include in this section full data on range, median, and mode MICs and an account of the percentage of strains inhibited at each concentration, would require many tables. We have therefore compromised by recording the median MIC of various cephalosporins for most organisms, and extended the data in parts where it was thought particularly necessary. It should also be noted that susceptibility varies geographically and temporally.

Antibacterial activity data

As discussed in the previous paragraph, in order to compare the activity of the cephalosporins against a variety of organisms, the MIC values expressed in the following tables are the median MICs for the strains tested by each worker quoted.

Tables 4 and 5 show the activity of parenterally- and orally-administered cephalosporins against Gram-positive cocci. In general the 'newer' cephalosporins tend to be slightly less active than cephalothin and cephaloridine. There is little difference between the MIC values for β-lactamase-producing and non-producing strains of *Staph. aureus* emphasising the point made in the earlier section on mechanisms of resistance (see under heading Beta-lactamases, this Chapter). Gram-positive β-lactamases have relatively little activity against cephalosporins compared with their activity against penicillins.

Str. faecalis is generally resistant to cephalosporins. In Figure 8 the

Table 5 Activity of orally-administered cephalosporins against Gram-positive cocci

| Organism | MIC (μg/ml) for 50% of strains | | |
	Cephalexin	Cephradine	Cefaclor
Staph. aureus (penicillin-sensitive)	1.5	1.0	1.5 6.0[30]*
Str. pyogenes	0.5	0.5	0.5
Str. pneumoniae	1.0	0.5	0.5
Str. faecalis	100	50	50

*.β -lactamase-producing strains – reference 30
Data from reference 29 except where stated otherwise

Table 4 Activity of some parenterally-administered cephalosporins against Gram-positive cocci

Organism	MIC (µg/ml) for 50% of strains tested						
	Cephalothin	Cephaloridine	Cefazolin	Cefamandole	Cefuroxime	Fefoxitin	Cefotaxime
Staph. aureus							
*Blac–	0.1[23]	0.19[25]	0.3[25]	0.1[23]	0.2[23]	2.5[525]	1.0[27]
**Blac+	0.3[24]			0.4[24]	0.1[23]	1.6[23]	1.0[27]
Staph. epidermidis	0.1[23]	–	0.2[23]	0.1[23]	–	1.6[23]	0.8[28]
	0.2[24]			0.2[24]	–		
Strept. pyogenes	0.19[25]	0.19[25]	0.19[25]	0.03[26]	–	0.78[25]	0.008[27]
Strept. pneumoniae	0.32[26]	0.2[26]	0.4[26]	0.4[26]	–	–	–
Strept. faecalis	50[26]	8[26]	12.5[23]	25[23]	–	25[23]	2.0[27]
							100[28]

Superscript numbers indicate references

* Non-β-lactamase-producing strains
** β'-lactamase-producing strains

Antibiotics and Chemotherapy

mode MIC of group D streptococci is compared with that of streptococci of groups A, B, C and G.

Table 6 shows the activity of nine cephalosporins against *H. influenzae*. Here it can be seen that β-lactamase has a role to play in the resistance of *H. influenzae* to cephalosporins. The MICs of enzyme-sensitive cephalosporins for β-lactamase-producing strains are approximately 4 times greater than those for β-lactamase non-producers. The enzyme-resistant cephalosporins – cefamandole, cefuroxime, cefoxitin and

Table 6   Activity of cephalosporins against *Haemophilus influenzae*

| Cephalosporin | MIC (μg/ml) *for* Haemophilus influenzae (50% of strains) | |
	β-lactamase producers	Non-β-lactamase producers
Cephalothin	6.0[31]	0.4[33] 1.0[34ɸ]
Cephaloridine·	16.0[31]	4.0[33] 1.56[34ɸ]
Cefazolin	12.0[31]	
Cephalexin	25.0[31]	4.0[33] 12.5[34ɸ]
Cephradine	48.0[31]	10.0[35]
Cefamandole	0.75[31]	0.2[33] 0.19[34ɸ]
Cefuroxime	0.5[32]	0.5[32]
Cefoxitin	3.0[31] 4.0[32]	2.0[32] 2.0[34ɸ]
Cefotaxime	0.1[32]	0.1[32] 0.004[27]

Superscript numbers indicate references

[34ɸ]   Results from 100 strains of *H. influenzae* (β-lactamase production not tested

[27]   Included 2/26 β-lactamase producing strains

cefotaxime – show equally good activity *in vitro* against β-lactamase-producing and non-producing strains of *H. influenzae*.

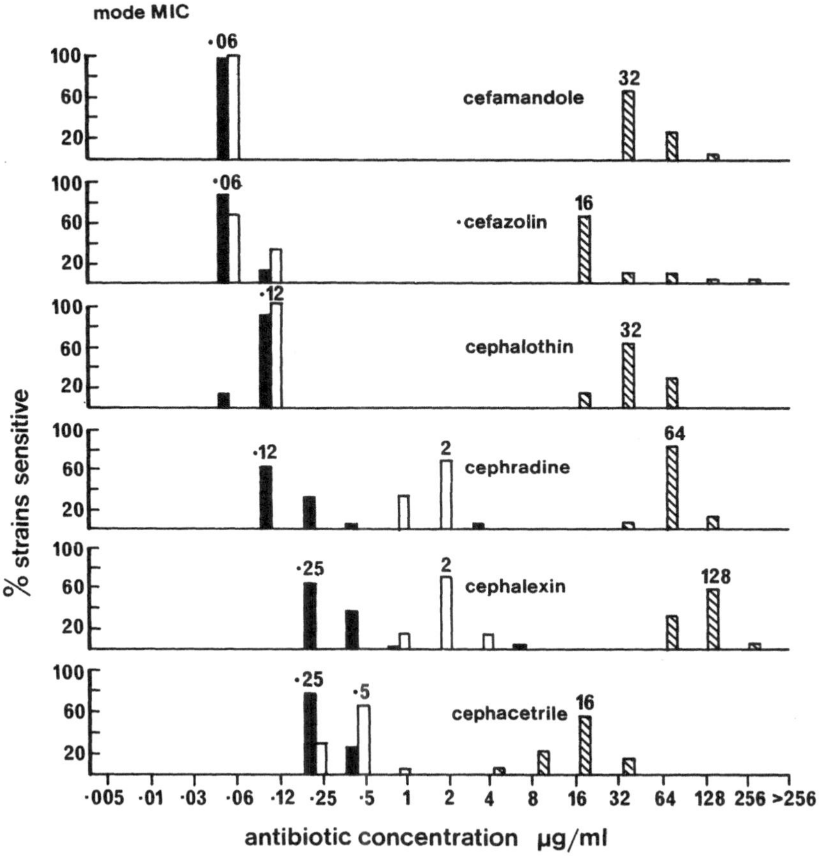

mode MIC

% strains sensitive

cefamandole

·cefazolin

cephalothin

cephradine

cephalexin

cephacetrile

antibiotic concentration μg/ml

Figure 8 Mode MIC of streptococci to 6 cephalosporins

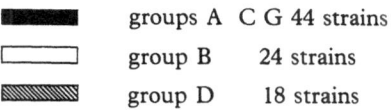

groups A C G 44 strains

group B   24 strains

group D   18 strains

Table 7 shows the range of MICs of some cephalosporins for β-lactamase-producing and non-producing strains of *H. influenzae.*

Tables 8 and 9 show the activity of parenterally- and orally-administered cephalosporins against aerobic Gram-negative bacilli. Here the effects of the enzyme stability of the newer cephalosporins can be seen most clearly. Table 10 shows the range and mode MICs of β-

Table 7   The range (and mode) of the MICs in μg/ml of ampicillin, cefoxitin and five cephalosporins for two groups of *H. influenzae*

Antibiotic	Ampicillin sensitive strains		β-lactamase producers	
Ampicillin	0.5		1–16	
Cefoxitin	1–16	(4)	2–4	(2)
Cefazolin	0.5–16		2–16	(16)
Cephaloridine	1–32	(2)	2–16	(4)
Cefuroxime	0.25–2	(0.5)	0.5–1	(0.5)
Cefamandole	0.12–2	(0.05)	0.25–2	(0.05)
Cefotaxime	0.003–0.06	(0.015)	0.003–0.03	(0.007–0.015)

lactamase stable cephalosporins for multi-resistant Gram-negative bacilli.

Table 11 shows the activity of selected cephalosporins against anaerobes. Cefoxitin has been found to be more active than cefamandole and other cephalosporins tested against strains of *Bacteroides fragilis.* Many strains of *B. fragilis* are β-lactamase producers but their resistance to β-lactam antibiotics appears to be reliant not only on β-lactamase production but also on the possession of a permeability barrier to β-lactam antibiotics. Cefotaxime is also active against some strains of *B. fragilis,* but in common with other cephalosporins, except cefoxitin, it is susceptible to β-lactamases produced by these organisms. Cefoxitin is resistant to hydrolysis by β-lactamases produced by all the subspecies of *B. fragilis* tested.

Table 12 shows the MICs for three different groups of *B. fragilis* strains. Strains sensitive to low concentrations of ampicillin (i.e. β-lactamase non-producers) are also sensitive to low concentrations of other β-lactam antibiotics. For an intermediate group with sensitivities to ampicillin ranging from 16–64 μg/ml, cefoxitin was the most active cephalosporin, followed by cefotaxime and cefuroxime. Against a group of highly ampicillin-resistant strains, only cefoxitin was active; the other cephalosporins tested were destroyed by β-lactamases produced by *B. fragilis.* Only one resistant strain failed to produce β-lactamase and its resistance was presumed to be due to a permeability barrier.

Against *Clostridium* spp. cefoxitin has activity similar to, or slightly less than, cefazolin, cephalothin and cefamandole. With the exception of

Table 8 Activity of some parenterally-administered cephalosporins against aerobic Gram-negative bacilli

Organism	MIC (μg/ml) for 50% of strains tested						
	Cephalothin	Cephaloridine	Cefazolin	Cefamandole	Cefuroxime	Cefoxitin	Cefotaxime
E. coli	50[23] 2.5[24]	2[37]	12.5[23] 1.6[38]	6.2[23] 0.8[24]	6.2[23]	12.5[23]	0.07[38] 0.06[27]
Klebsiella	3.1[23] 6.3[24]	3[37]	3.1[23] 5.5[38]	0.4[23] 1.6[24]	1.6[23]	1.6[23]	0.08[38] 0.06[27]
Enterobacter	R[23] R[24]	R[37]	40[38] R[23]	3.1[23] 3.1[24]	6.2[23]	50[23]	30[38] 0.06[27]
Citrobacter	24[23]	–	R[23] 40[38]	0.2[23]	3.1[23]	6.2[23]	2.4[38]
Serratia	R[23] R[24]	R[37]	R[23] 40[38]	R[24] R[23]	50[23]	50[23]	0.85[38] 0.06[27]
Proteus mirabilis	6.2[23] 6.3[24]	2[37]	6.2[23] 9.0[38]	1.6[23] 1.6[24]	1.6[23]	3.1[23]	0.03[38] 0.06[27]
Proteus (indole+)	R[23] R[24]	R[37]	40[38] R[23]	3.1[22] 3.1[24]	25[23]	6.2[23]	0.75[38] 0.06[27]
Providencia	R[23]	R[37]	40[38]	12.5[23]	25[23]	6.2[23]	0.12[27]
Salmonella spp. typhi paratyphi A	6.3[23] 0.8[36] 5.0[36]		1.7[38] 0.75[36] 2.0[36]	3.1[23] 0.19[36] 1.0[36]		1.6[23]	0.12[38] 0.06[27]
Shigella	25[23]			1.6[23]		6.3[23]	

Superscript numbers indicate references
R̄ =>64 μg/ml

Table 9 Activity of orally-administered cephalosporins against aerobic Gram-negative rods

Organism	MIC (μg/ml) for 50% of strains		
	Cephalexin	Cephradine	Cefaclor
E. coli	4[37]	8[29]	12[30]
			4[29]
Klebsiella	3[37]	6[29]	6[30]
			4[29]
Enterobacter	32[37]	50[29]	4[29]
Citrobacter	–	–	–
Serratia	R[37]	–	–
Proteus mirabilis	4[37]	20[29]	4[29]
Proteus (indole +)	50[37]	R[29]	32[30]
			R[29]
Salmonella (spp.)			
typhi	2.5[36]		0.3[36]
paratyphi A	10.0[36]		1.0[36]
Shigella			12[30]

Superscripts indicate references
R = >64μg/ml

B. fragilis, benzyl penicillin is generally more active against most anaerobes than the cephalosporins and cefoxitin.

Until recently *Ps. aeruginosa* has remained unscathed by the cephalosporin group of antibiotics but recent modifications of the cephalosporin molecule have resulted in new agents which have antipseudomonal activity.

Cefotaxime when tested[43] against 245 clinical isolates of *Ps. aeruginosa* gave MIC values ranging between those of azlocillin and carbenicillin. Against 31 strains of gentamicin-resistant *Ps. aeruginosa* the MICs ranged from 4μg/ml–64μg/ml with a mode MIC value of 16μg/ml.

Cefsulodin is a new cephalosporin with activity directed primarily against *Ps. aeruginosa* and Gram-positive cocci. It is less active than other cephalosporins against Gram-negative bacilli other than *Ps. aeruginosa*. This high antipseudomonal activity is thought to be related partly to a high affinity of the agent for the penicillin-binding proteins in the pseudomonas' cell membrane and partly to the resistance of the drug

Table 10 Range and mode MICs of β-lactamase-stable cephalosporins and cefoxitin against multi-resistant Gram-negative bacilli

Organism	No. of strains	Cefotaxime	Cefamandole	Cefuroxime	Cefoxitin
Pseudomonas aeruginosa	31	4 – R (16)	R (R)	R (R)	R (R)
Serratia	13	0.25– 32 (1)	R (R)	32– R (R)	16– R (R)
Citrobacter	7	0.12– 2 (1)	32– R (R)	4– R (R)	R (R)
Klebsiella	26	0.06– 32 (0.06)	0.5– R (R)	1– R (2)	2– R (2)
Providencia	33	0.06– 2 (0.06)	0.25– R (1)	0.25– R (2)	0.25– R (2)
Enterobacter	34	0.06– 32 (1)	1– R (R)	2– R (R)	2– R (R)
Acinetobacter	22	0.06– R (16)	0.5– R (R)	2– R (R)	2– R (R)
Alkaligenes	11	0.25– R (R)	8– R (R)	16– R (R)	0.5– R (R)

All bacterial strains were resistant to ampicillin and gentamicin
Modified from Drasar et al.[32]
R = >64 ug/ml

Table 11 Activity of four cephalosporins against anaerobes

Organism tested	MIC for 50% of strains (µg/ml)			
	Cephalothin	Cefazolin	Cefamandole	Cefoxitin
Bacteroides fragilis	64[39]	50[39]	30[21]	8[39]
	50[23]	50[23]	64[39]	4[25]
			50[23]	
Bacteroides spp. (other than *fragilis*)	4[39]	1[39]	2[39]	2[39]
			0.5[42]	
Fusobacterium	0.25[39]	0.25[39]	0.25[39]	0.5[39]
Campylobacter	4.0[39]*	8[39]	8[39]	32[39]
	100[40]*			75[40]
Clostridium welchii other spp.	0.75[39]	0.5[39]	0.5[39]	0.75[39]
			0.5[42]	
			0.12[42]	
Peptococcus	0.25[39]	0.25[39]	0.5[39]	0.25[39]
			0.12[42]	
Peptostreptococcus	0.25[39]	0.25[39]	0.25[39]	0.25[39]
Actinomyces	2[39]	0.5[39]	0.25[39]	0.5[39]
Eubacterium	0.25[39]	0.25[39]	0.25[39]	0.5[39]
Lactobacillus	4[39]	2[39]	8[39]	10[39]
Bifidobacterium	4[39]	1[39]	0.5[39]	4[39]
Propionibacterium	0.25[39]	0.25[39]	0.25[39]	0.25[39]
			0.12[42]	
Veillonella	0.25[39]	0.25[39]	0.25[39]	0.75[39]
Eikenella corrodens	12[41]	6[41]	12[41]	1[41]

Superscript numbers indicate references

[39]* 6/8 *Camp. fetus* 2/8 *Camp. sputorum*

[40]* *Camp. fetus* subsp. *jejuni*

to pseudomonal β-lactamases[45]. Cefsulodin tested against 180 clinical isolates of *Ps. aeruginosa* inhibited 90% of strains at a concentration of 16 µg/ml or less, whereas only 10% of the strains were inhibited by the same concentration of carbenicillin. 16 µg/ml is a concentration that can be achieved in the serum by normal dosage of this antibiotic[45].

Table 12 Range and mode MICs in μg/ml of ampicillin, cefoxitin and 4 cephalosporins for 3 groups of *Bacteroides fragilis* (mode MIC in parenthesis)

Antibiotic	Sensitive strains 8	Standard strains 4	Resistant strains 5
Ampicillin	0.25–4 (1)	16–64 (32)	128 (128)
Cefoxitin	1–2 (1)	2–16 (4)	8–64 (8)
Cefazolin	0.5–8 (2)	16–128 (32)	128 (128)
Cefuroxime	0.5–4 (2)	4–128 (8)	128 (128)
Cefamandole	0.5–4 (2)	16–128 (64)	128 (128)
	0.25–8 (2)	4–128 (8)	128 (128)

After Drasar et al.[32]

Reproduced with permission from Journal of Antimicrobial Chemotherapy

Two other antipseudomonal cephalosporins are at present under investigation – Ly 127935 (6059-S) (Lilly) and cefoperazone. The chemical structures of these compounds have been shown in an earlier section (see Figure 1). Cefoperazone is a 'true' cephalosporin, whereas 6059-S is the first of a new class of β-lactam antibiotics, a 1-oxacephalosporin, with oxygen in place of sulphur in the β-lactam nucleus. Both compounds appear to have similar characteristics *in vitro*; they are active against *Ps. aeruginosa* and also against other Gram-negative bacilli including *Proteus* spp., *Enterobacter* and *Serratia*. Neither compound shows particular activity against Gram-positive cocci. 6059-S is active against *Bacteroides fragilis* subsp. *fragilis* but cefoperazone is not. Both compounds are very stable to hydrolysis by β-lactamases (Table 13).

Table 13   The range and mode of the MICs of 4 cephalosporins, gentamicin and carbenicillin for 65 strains of *Pseudomonas aeruginosa*

Antibiotic	MIC (μg/ml)	
	Range	Mode
Cefotaxime	4–128	16
Cefsulodin	0.5–128	4
Cefoperazone	0.5– 32	4
Ly127935(6059-S)	4–128	32
Gentamicin	2–128	8
Carbenicillin	0.5–128	128

(Williams, R. J. and Williams, J. D. : unpublished data)

PHARMACOLOGY

The relative advantage of one cephalosporin over another may depend primarily on differences in pharmacokinetic characteristics. Pharmacokinetic features which are considered to be advantageous include good absorption from different sites, high serum concentrations, low serum protein binding, long serum half-life and a large apparent volume of distribution. These aspects will be considered in the following sections.

Absorption

Orally-absorbed cephalosporins
Oral absorption of cephalexin and cephradine and cefaclor result in peak serum concentrations ranging from 18–48 μg/ml (Table 14). Twenty-four hour urine recovery is almost 100% indicating the completeness of absorption of the drugs from the gastro-intestinal tract.

Table 14   Comparison of pharmacokinetics of orally-absorbed cephalosporins

Cephalosporin	Dose (oral route)	Mean peak serum concentration (μg/ml)	Time of peak post-dose (min)	Ref.
Cephalexin	500 mg	27.6	81	46
Cephradine	500 mg	18.0	40	47
Cefaclor	500 mg	12.4	60	48
	1 g	48.3	60	49

Oral administration with food does not affect the extent of absorption but does result in a delay in onset of absorption, lower peak serum concentrations and more sustained blood levels.

In terms of pharmacokinetics, there appears to be little difference between the available oral cephalosporins (see Tables 14 and 15).

Parenterally-administered cephalosporins
The oral absorption of cephalosporins manufactured for parenteral use is low, but all of them can be given intravenously or intramuscularly. They are all well-absorbed after intramuscular administration but pain at the injection site is common and most pronounced with cephalothin and cephapirin which should be restricted preferably to intravenous use. Cephradine, which is available for parenteral and oral administration, is better absorbed after oral than after intramuscular administration and the latter may result in unpredictable serum concentrations[47].

Intravenous administration of cephalosporins quite commonly results in thrombophlebitis but studies of this aspect have produced highly conflicting results reflecting differences in the methods of administration and the type of infusion apparatus used.

Cephaloridine reaches peak serum concentrations approximately twice those of cephalothin after similar doses and is excreted more

Table 15 Comparison of some pharmacokinetic properties of cephalosporins and related compounds

Cephalosporin	Peak serum concentration (µg/ml) after stated dose	Urinary excretion in stated time (h)	Serum half-life[ϕ] (min)	% Protein binding[ϕ]	Volume[ϕ] distribution (1)*
Cephaloridine	22 500 mg IM	80% in 24[51]	48–94	10–31	27
Cephalothin	10 500 mg IM	64% in 4[51]	28–50	62–79	22
Cefazolin	54 1 g IM	80% in 24[52]	69–120	74–76	10
Cefamandole	31 1 g IM	70% in 8[53]	34–54	74	22
Cefuroxime	33 1 g IM	85% in 8[54]	62–120	33	22
Cefoxitin	22 1 g IM	80% in 2[25]	42–59	65–75	8
Cephradine	see Table 14	100% in 24[51]	32–62	6–20	22
Cephalexin	see Table 14	100% in 24[51]	36–54	10–15	18

ϕ   Data reproduced from K. E. Andersson (1978). On the pharmacokinetics of cephalosporin antibiotics, *Scand. J. Infect. Dis.* (*Suppl.*), **13**, 37, with permission

*   Some of the data were originally expressed as 1/1.73 but have been converted to 1 for comparability

Superscript numbers indicate references

slowly, detectable activity being present in the serum 8 h after the dose (Table 15).

Comparative data for cefazolin, cefamandole, cefuroxime and cefoxitin are shown in Table 15. Cefoxitin is much more rapidly excreted than other cephalosporins, 80% of a 1 g dose being recovered in the urine after 2 h. With cefazolin, cefamandole and cefuroxime, 70–90% of the dose is excreted by 8 h.

Both one- and two-compartment models have been applied to the pharmacokinetics of cephalosporins. In a study of cefamandole[50], computer analysis of serum antibiotic concentrations against time fitted with great accuracy a two-compartment open model. This model leads to the assumption that the antibiotic is injected into a central compartment which corresponds roughly to the blood volume; an equilibrium is rapidly reached between this central compartment and a larger peripheral compartment corresponding to all the different tissues into which the antibiotic diffuses. Cefamandole is eliminated by passing from the central compartment into the urine. The initial phase is characterised by distribution of antibiotic with a rapid fall in serum concentrations and it is followed by an elimination phase with a slower exponential decline in serum concentrations. It is thought that this type of model is generally applicable to all cephalosporins.

Distribution

Although the achievable serum concentrations of an antibiotic are used as a means of predicting the likely therapeutic response, it is probably only the free, non-protein-bound fraction of this serum concentration which is antibacterially active. Thus the degree of protein binding is important and will affect the extra-vascular concentration of the antibiotic. The binding of various cephalosporins to serum proteins differs, as shown in Table 15. In addition the degree of binding of one cephalosporin varies between the serum proteins of different animal species.

An antibiotic with a long serum half-life may in part offset the negative effect of a high degree of protein binding. The serum half-lives of different cephalosporins are shown in Table 15. Other factors which affect the extravascular antibiotic concentration are the concentration gradient from plasma to extracellular fluid, the lipid solubility and the state of ionisation of the antibiotic.

The apparent volume of distribution gives information on the quotient between the amount of antibiotic in the body and the serum concentration at a certain time. The apparent volumes of distribution of various cephalosporins are shown in Table 15.

Although a large volume of distribution has been considered a favourable characteristic when choosing a cephalosporin for clinical use, this does not give any information about the distribution of the antibiotic to a particular organ or tissue. Some areas of the body, e.g. muscle, bone, synovial and interstitial fluid, are more readily accessible to intravascular antibiotic via aqueous pores in the capillary endothelium. Other areas, e.g. CSF, brain, eye, intestine and prostate, do not apparently have such pores and penetration of cephalosporins into these sites depends on their ability to cross lipid membranes. Thus penetration may vary considerably between cephalosporins depending on their lipid solubility.

Distribution of cephalosporins to various parts of the body
(a) *Bone* Cephalothin penetration into cortical bone was studied in 105 patients undergoing arthroplasty of the hip. Osseous tissue concentrations one hour after a 1 g intravenous dose ranged from 0.9–17.5μg/g (mean 3.8μg/g) while the mean serum concentration collected at the same time was 11.9μg/ml. However, the authors found that there was no consistent relationship between cortical bone concentration and serum concentration[55].

Cefamandole has been studied in a similar group of patients[56]. A single 2 g intravenous dose resulted in bone concentrations averaging 8.5μg/g but if this dose was followed by a 2 g intravenous infusion perioperatively, bone concentrations were raised to 61 μg/g.

(b) *Tissue, fluid and inflammatory exudate* A skin abrasion technique was used to measure inflammatory exudate concentrations of cefazolin and cephaloridine in patients undergoing elective surgery[57]. Concentrations of both cephalosporins in inflammatory exudate were found to be almost identical to serum concentrations and considerably higher than wound concentrations. In all three sites, cefazolin achieved higher concentrations than cephaloridine when given in the same dosage.

Ascitic fluid concentrations of cephalosporins were studied in dogs[58]. Concentrations of cefazolin and cephaloridine were significantly higher than cephalothin and cefamandole but the serum concentrations were also found to be higher for the two former agents and the percentage penetration was not significantly different among the four cephalosporins. There was appreciable binding of cephalosporins to ascitic fluid.

Also in dogs, interstitial fluid concentrations of cefaclor were found to be lower than serum concentrations during the 4 hours post-dose[59].

In a comparison of cefamandole and cephalothin as prophylactic agents for open-heart surgery, tissue concentrations of cefamandole were always greater than those of cephalothin when administered in the same dose[60].

Table 16   Cephalosporins in cerebrospinal fluid

Cephalosporin	Concentration in (μg/ml):			Subjects	Ref.
	CSF	*Serum*	*CSF/Serum %*		
Cephalothin	0.16			Humans with normal meninges	63
Cephalothin			1.8	Dogs with experi-mental meningitis	64
Cephalothin	0.16–0.31	10–80		Human meningitis	63
Cephalothin	0.15–46.5		7–88	Human meningococcal meningitis	65
Cephalothin			5.6	Human meningitis	66
Cephaloridine			25	Rabbits with meningitis	67
Cephaloridine			1.4	Dogs with experi-mental meningitis	64
Cephaloridine	0.4–5.6	7–21		Acute bacterial meningitis; human	68
Cephaloridine			10.9	Human meningitis	66
Cefamandole			4	Humans without active meningitis	69
Cefamandole			23	Humans with active meningitis	69
Cefazolin	0.62	40–320		Humans with normal CSF	70
Cefazolin	0.65–5.0			Humans with meningitis or post-neurosurgery	70
Cefoxitin	0.63	60		Humans with normal meninges	25
Cefoxitin	0.63	60		Normal humans having single dose	71
Cefoxitin	2.9	94		Normal humans having multiple doses	71

(c) *Bronchial secretions* Specimens of bronchial secretions were collected from patients during episodes of bronchopulmonary infection from patients receiving intravenous cefoxitin. Following an intravenous infusion cefoxitin passes progressively into the bronchial mucus. The average concentration of cefoxitin in bronchial secretions was greater than 1.5 µg/ml and reached 5 µg/ml in a few patients[61].

(d) *Eye* Studies have shown that cephalothin and cephaloridine reach therapeutic concentrations against Gram-positive organisms in the primary aqueous humour of the eye[62]. Intramuscular administration of cefamandole resulted in no detectable antibiotic in the primary aqueous humour but following 1 and 2 g intravenous doses the aqueous humour concentrations ranged from 0.33–0.14 µg/ml, and 1.26–0.73 µg/ml during 5 hours post-dose respectively. With respect to common Gram-positive pathogens in serious eye infections, cefamandole reached potentially efficacious levels but therapeutic levels against Gram-negative organisms were rarely reached[62].

(e) *Cerebrospinal fluid* Penetration of various cephalosporins into the CSF is shown in Table 16.

Metabolism
Some cephalosporins undergo metabolic degradation in the body. Cephalothin is metabolised to desacetylcephalothin, probably in the liver and kidneys. Cephapirin and cephacetrile are also desacetylated. The desacetyl derivatives retain some antibacterial activity but this is considerably lower than that of the parent compound. However, this will affect the results of microbiological assays used in determination of cephalothin concentrations. In order to distinguish between the metabolites and the parent compound, alternative assay methods must be employed, e.g. HPLC.

Cefoxitin is metabolised to the descarbamyl form but only to an insignificant amount *in vivo*.

Excretion
The main route of excretion of all cephalosporins is via the kidney. More than 90% of cephaloridine is excreted by glomerular filtration, whereas cephalothin and cephacetrile are excreted mainly by tubular secretion. Other cephalosporins are excreted by both methods to varying extents. In renal insufficiency the elimination of all cephalosporins is impaired but the effect of impairment varies with different cephalosporins depending on their particular method of renal excretion.

The major part of a dose of any cephalosporin is excreted within 24 hours of administration and for several cephalosporins more than

50% of the dose is excreted within 6 hours of administration.

The only other recognised route of excretion of cephalosporins is via the biliary system. Biliary concentrations of cephalosporins have been studied by many workers but it is difficult to compare results for different members of the cephalosporin group since the studies vary considerably in dose and route of administration of the antibiotic and in the types of patients studied. The majority of studies have been done on patients undergoing cholecystectomy or with T-tubes *in situ* and there are no data available on biliary excretion in normal humans.

Cephalothin bile concentrations in patients undergoing cholecystectomy were found to be approximately the same as serum concentrations one hour after a 1 g intravenous dose[72]. Ratzan and colleagues[52] compared the excretion of cefazolin and cephaloridine with cephalothin in patients undergoing cholecystectomy. Following a single 1 g dose and in the absence of cystic duct obstruction, the mean antibiotic concentrations in gall bladder bile were 17, 7 and 1 μg/ml for cefazolin, cephaloridine and cephalothin respectively. But where there was cystic duct obstruction, none of these cephalosporins was detectable in appreciable amounts in gall bladder bile.

Cefazolin has been found by other workers[73][74] to be well excreted in bile although concentrations are always considerably lower in the presence of duct obstruction. However, cefamandole is reported to reach concentrations 50 times those of cefazolin and 400 times those of cephalothin in the gall bladder bile of patients with non-obstructive cholecystitis and cholelithiasis. In gall bladder tissue also, concentrations of cefamandole and cefazolin were much greater than those of cephalothin[56].

In patients given multiple doses of cephalexin prior to cholecystectomy, high antibiotic concentrations were found in gall bladder bile in those with radiologically-functioning gall bladders and even where the gall bladder was non-functioning, measurable amounts of cephalexin were present[75].

Cefoxitin is well-excreted in bile, reaching peak concentrations 2–4 h after administration, but these are again considerably reduced in the presence of cystic duct obstruction. However, concentrations of 26 μg/ml and 25 μg/ml in gall bladder tissue have been reported in the absence and presence of cystic duct obstruction respectively[25].

In studies in dogs, cefaclor appears to be actively excreted in bile at concentrations more than sufficient to be effective against susceptible pathogens[59].

The biliary route of excretion has received considerable study because of the possibility of using cephalosporins in the treatment of biliary tract infections. This will be discussed in a later section.

TOXICITY

Allergic reactions

Our understanding of the nature and significance of immune responsiveness to β-lactam antibiotics is limited. Both penicillins and
cephalosporins stimulate in man and experimental animals a specific
immunological response but this is not paralleled by allergic responsiveness and adverse reactions of a hypersensitivity nature are relatively
uncommon. Humans develop allergic reactions to cephalosporins and
their sera contain antibodies detectable by passive haemagglutination
with red blood cells coated with cephalothin[76]; the antibodies appear to
be IgE in nature. Penicillin-allergic patients have been shown to have a
raised total IgE when measured by radio-immunoassay or radioactive
single radial diffusion techniques[77].

Levine *et al.*[78] found that 13% of a group of randomly selected
individuals had penicilloyl-specific antibodies of IgG class. The one
condition in which this antibody seems to be of aetiological significance
is haemolytic anaemia, a rare complication of high dose intravenous
therapy. Of the same random group, 97% had specific antibodies to
penicillins and cephalosporins of the IgM class. These are probably of
little clinical significance but may be important in some late-developing
rashes.

To what extent do patients with penicillin allergy cross react with
cephalosporins? There is definitely some cross-reactivity but this is
difficult to quantify[76]. A survey by Dash[79] suggested that 91–94% of
patients with a history of penicillin allergy did not react to cephalosporins. The probable clinical outcome of therapy with a cephalosporin
in a patient allergic to benzyl penicillin differs in different individuals
and it is likely to be largely predicted by skin tests[80]. Cross-allergy in
penicillin-sensitive patients has occasionally been observed in treatment
with cephaloglycin and cephalexin but the newer cephalosporins appear
to be only rarely cross-allergic with penicillins.

Allergic reactions are possible with all cephalosporin preparations but
the incidence of cephalosporin allergy is less than that of penicillin
allergy[81]. In addition, not all cephalosporin allergies are found in
patients who are penicillin-allergic; some are due to independent
sensitisation. For example, allergic reactions to cephalothin and
cephaloridine have occurred in the absence of known history of
penicillin allergy. Some individuals develop an allergic reaction soon
after the start of cephalosporin therapy, which suggests either cross-
reaction or prior cephalosporin sensitisation. Others develop a reaction
some days later, indicating a primary cephalosporin allergy[78].

Available evidence suggests that the overall rate of hypersensitivity to cephalosporins is not greater than 10% and does not appear to be related to dose or duration of treatment. However, in one volunteer study the rate of adverse reactions was very much higher. Sanders and colleagues[82] administered cephalothin to 15 healthy volunteers and cephapirin to another 15, in doses up to 2 g four times daily by rapid intravenous infusion. The dosage schedule was planned for 30 days but the incidence of adverse reactions was so high that the study was curtailed. Results of skin tests with penicillin and search for anti-penicillin haemagglutinating antibodies were not suggestive of pre-existing penicillin hypersensitivity. There were few immediate reactions to skin tests with cephalothin or cephapirin and there was a similar lack of delayed hypersensitivity reactions on skin testing. This suggested either that the antibodies which evoked the illness were not native cephalothin or cephapirin or that the illness was not mediated by IgE. The diagnosis of a hypersensitivity reaction was supported primarily by clinical and pathological findings and the authors have concluded that prolonged high dose intravenous therapy may have precipitated the adverse reactions. These results are unusual[82].

There is a tendency to eosinophilia in patients receiving cephalosporin therapy and skin rashes occasionally occur.

Nephrotoxicity
Administration of high doses of cephaloridine or cephalothin to experimental animals damages the proximal cells of the kidney tubules, resulting in acute tubular necrosis. The degree of damage, and the dose at which damage occurs, depends on the animal species. The kidney tissue concentrations associated with nephrotoxicity are not known but it is probable that tubular transport mechanisms are involved[83].

Cephaloridine is not secreted by the kidney to any significant degree (95% is filtered through the glomerulus) but it is still actively transported into the proximal tubule cells where it exerts its toxic effect. This effect can be prevented by pre-administration of probenicid or certain other organic anions which inhibit renal cortical cephaloridine uptake[84]. It is possible that cephalothin, which is also secreted by the organic anion transport system may protect the kidney against cephaloridine toxicity by preventing its uptake by the proximal tubule[84].

In an analysis of 36 cases of possible cephalosporin-associated nephrotoxicity, Foord[83] showed that patients who developed renal failure during cephaloridine therapy had peak serum concentrations in the range 130–360 μg/ml. Nephrotoxicity does not occur if peak serum concentrations are maintained in the range 20–80 μg/ml, and concentrations greater than 100 μg/ml are unnecessary and unsafe.

Foord[83] found that 71% of cephaloridine-treated patients and 55% of cephalothin patients who developed nephrotoxicity received excessive doses which were not adjusted to allow for impaired renal function. In most cases, the acute tubular necrosis was reversible when therapy ceased.

There is growing evidence that cephalothin can be nephrotoxic under certain circumstances. Cephalothin differs from cephaloridine in that 80% of the drug is secreted through the tubular wall and only 20% is filtered through the glomerulus. 35–40% of the circulating antibiotic is metabolised to desacetylcephalothin. Information on toxic serum concentrations comparable with those for cephaloridine is not available.

Prior to renal failure many of the patients showed signs of tubular 'irritation' resulting in hyaline casts, cells, and sometimes protein in the urine. Stopping therapy at this stage aids rapid recovery of the tubular cells. In an attempt to determine the effect of cephaloridine on normal kidneys, Linsell et al.[85] examined urine from bronchitics receiving 6 g/day cephaloridine. They found that hyaline cast production increased during treatment and returned to normal after the drug was withdrawn.

There are a number of factors, apart from the dose of cephaloridine or cephalothin, which may affect the development of renal toxicity and in any study of patients developing nephrotoxicity it is often difficult to separate these factors and determine which of them is responsible. Contributory factors include:

(a) Age of patient. (Renal clearance decreases considerably over 50 years of age.)
(b) Severe sepsis
(c) Hypotension
(d) Congestive cardiac failure
(e) Haemorrhage
(f) Dehydration
(g) Surgery
(h) Concurrent treatment with diuretics, particularly frusemide
(i) Concurrent treatment with other antibiotics.

There has been considerable debate on the interpretation of data on the nephrotoxicity of combinations of aminoglycosides and cephalosporins. Both aminoglycosides and cephalosporins are known to be potentially nephrotoxic antibiotics. The general trend of results from therapeutic trials and case reports suggests that aminoglycosides and cephalosporins, particularly gentamicin and cephalothin, may be synergistic in their toxic effects[86] [87]. Wade et al.[88] carried out a prospective randomised double-blind trial to compare the incidence of nephrotoxicity in patients with suspected sepsis treated with cephalothin and gentamicin, or cephalothin and tobramycin, or methicillin and gentamicin, or methicillin and tobramycin. Nephrotoxicity developed in 25.5% of patients whose regimen included cephalothin but in only 7% of patients who received methicillin with their aminglycoside. This difference was statistically significant and suggests that cephalothin was the more nephrotoxic agent.

However, efforts to examine the effects of cephalosporin and aminoglycoside combinations in animals have produced conflicting results. Some workers have found that gentamicin and cephaloridine given separately to rats in doses far exceeding normal human dosage gave rise to proximal tubular necrosis. However, these effects were not produced by doses giving blood levels of antibiotic comparable to those seen in man[89]. Dellinger *et al.*[90] administered gentamicin and cephalothin to rats in a 'chequerboard' dosage regimen with gentamicin doses ranging from 6–50 mg/kg day $^{-1}$, and cephalothin from 200–800 mg/kg day $^{-1}$. They found no evidence of potentiation of gentamicin nephrotoxicity by cephalothin. On the contrary, at any given dose of gentamicin, renal tubular necrosis was significantly decreased by the simultaneous administration of cephalothin. But this protective effect was not seen if the doses of the two antibiotics were staggered by 6 hours.

It is difficult to assess the relevance of animal studies to man, especially when different animal species show different degrees of nephrotoxicity with the same cephalosporin. They appear to be contrary to the general observations of combined gentamicin and cephalosporin therapy in humans which are also much affected by the underlying conditions of the patients as discussed above.

In patients treated with cephalexin no impairment of renal function has been noted and cephalexin does not appear to aggravate pre-existing renal disease.

Parenterally-administered cephaglycin was found to be markedly more toxic in mice and rats than cephalothin or cephaloridine[91].

An association has been demonstrated between administration of a single large dose of cefazolin to rabbits and the appearance of focal renal injury[92]. The lesions were similar to those produced by cephaloridine but much higher doses of cefazolin were required to produce the lesions. The doses used were far higher than recommended for human use. When administered to rats on a long-term basis, the extent of renal injury produced by both cefazolin and cephaloridine was dose-dependent but cephaloridine was toxic at lower dose levels. However, the serum concentrations of cefazolin were approximately twice those of cephaloridine suggesting that peak serum levels alone are not the reason for the observed nephrotoxicity. There has been no evidence of nephrotoxicity in humans treated with cefazolin in doses up to 12 g/day.

Cefamandole appears in animal studies to be less nephrotoxic than cefazolin[93]. Similarly, in mice and rats, high doses of cefuroxime were not nephrotoxic although acute tubular necrosis did occur if frusemide was administered concurrently. Combined therapy with cefuroxime and an aminoglycoside lessened the nephrotoxic effect of the aminoglycoside[94].

Animal studies with cefoxitin failed to demonstrate nephrotoxicity and cefoxitin does not appear to be nephrotoxic when administered in moderate doses to patients with slightly impaired renal function. Concurrent treatment with frusemide does not prolong serum half-life or affect renal function[95].

Encephalopathy

Neurological disturbances such as those encountered with large doses of penicillin G can occur when high serum cephaloridine concentrations are reached. Murdoch[96] reported hallucinations and nystagmus occurring in two patients who were given 100 mg/day cephaloridine intrathecally, but the effects were not observed when the dose was reduced to 50 mg/day.

Cephaloridine given intravenously was found to be twice as toxic as cephalothin in the mouse and three times as toxic in the rat. Deaths occurred within a few minutes apparently as a result of central nervous system toxicity[91]. However, the doses were vastly in excess of those recommended for humans. In mice, 5 g/kg intravenous dose of cephalothin led to clonic convulsions with deaths occurring within 24 hours. Convulsions were not observed when cephalothin was given by other routes. When administered intracerebrally to mice, cephalothin had one fifteenth of the toxicity of benzyl penicillin[91].

Cephalexin may occasionally cause neurological disturbances in humans and very high concentrations may lead to convulsions and coma.

Encephalopathy has not been recorded with the newer cephalosporins.

Haematological abnormalities

Many of the cephalosporins will give a positive direct Coomb's test. This may interfere with cross-matching procedures but otherwise causes no ill effects. Cephalothin may cause an aggregation-type haemolytic anaemia. The antibiotic binds to red blood cells and in doing so aggregates serum proteins as well. In this condition either the IgG Coomb's or C_3 Coomb's test, or both, may be positive.

Other haematological effects are rare. Cephalothin may give rise to a prolongation of prothrombin time. There have been occasional reports of transient leucopaenia following treatment with cephaloridine[97], cephalothin[98] and cefoxitin[25]. Cephalothin-induced thrombocytopaenia, apparently due to binding of specific antibody to cephalothin-coated platelets, has been recorded[99].

Hepatotoxicity
Transient elevations of SGOT, SGPT and alkaline phosphatase have been noted during therapy with many of the cephalosporins, but no serious cases of hepatotoxicity have been reported.

Other toxic effects

Gastro-intestinal irritation
Diarrhoea, vomiting and abdominal cramps are the most frequent side effects of cephaloglycin therapy. Pruritis and moniliasis may also occur. Similar effects are seen with cephalexin and oral cephradine, but are less common.

Pain on administration
Many of the cephalosporins are very painful when injected intramuscularly and it may be necessary to dilute the injection with a local anaesthetic such as lignocaine. Thrombophlebitis at the site of intravenous injection is quite frequently reported.

Teratogenicity
Teratogenicity due to cephalosporins has not been recorded in animals or humans and these antibiotics can safely be used in the first trimester of pregnancy. No adverse effects such as haemolytic anaemia in newborn have been noted when mothers were given cephalosporins near term.

Cephalothin-induced meningitis
The development of bacterial meningitis in five patients who were receiving cephalothin for infections elswhere in the body gave rise to the suggestion that cephalothin treatment may induce bacterial meningitis[66]. This suggestion has since been discredited.

CLINICAL USES OF CEPHALOSPORINS

The cephalosporins are a group of antibiotics with antibacterial activity against many bacterial species. They are widely and increasingly used in the treatment of many types of infection. However, the precise place of each of the cephalosporins in the treatment of infections remains to be carefully defined in relation to the alternative antibiotics available. There are numerous reports in the literature of the use of individual compounds and this section is intended only as a survey of the possible role of cephalosporins in the treatment of infection.

Respiratory tract infections

Acute chest infections are most frequently caused by *Str. pneumoniae* and *H. influenzae*. *Str. pneumoniae* is sensitive to the cephalosporins, and cephalothin or cephaloridine may be used as alternatives to penicillin, but they are less effective and more expensive. The oral cephalosporin, cephalexin, does not penetrate well into sputum and is not recommended for the treatment of pneumococcal infections. The newer, β-lactamase resistant, cephalosporins are generally less active than cephaloridine and cephalothin against the Gram-positive cocci.

H. influenzae is only moderately sensitive to the cephalosporins although the newer agents, cefamandole, cefuroxime and cefotaxime have greater activity. Despite this, cephalosporins, including the oral agents have been used extensively in the treatment of acute exacerbations of chronic bronchitis with reported success. However, controlled trials are not available and the incidence of viral infections and the influence of self-limiting infections on the reported cure rates is not elucidated. There is little evidence to show that the cephalosporins are superior to ampicillin or co-trimoxazole.

In more severe pulmonary infections, especially those acquired in hospital, *Staph. aureus* and Gram-negative bacilli may be significant pathogens. Cephalothin and cephaloridine are satisfactory antistaphylococcal agents and generally better than the newer cephalosporins. However the drugs of choice in staphylococcal infections are usually cloxacillin, flucloxacillin and fucidin. The cephalosporins may have a role in the treatment of infection in penicillin-allergic patients.

Gram-negative pneumonia is often difficult to treat and the aminoglycosides probably take preference over the cephalosporins even when the infecting organism is cephalosporin-sensitive. In the future, the new antipseudomonal cephalosporins may play a useful role in the treatment of pneumonia caused by *Ps. aeruginosa*.

Cephalosporins are not indicated for mycoplasmal, chlamydial or fungal infections of the lung.

Urinary tract infections

The organisms responsible for urinary tract infections in domiciliary practice are usually susceptible to many antibacterial agents including ampicillin, sulphonamides, co-trimoxazole, nitrofurantoin, nalidixic acid and the cephalosporins. Since oral treatment is required cephalexin, cephradine and cefaclor are the relevant cephalosporins. These agents have been used successfully in the treatment of urinary tract infections and the choice between cephalosporins and other antibiotics for treating sensitive organisms is made on the basis of patient factors such as hypersensitivity and other side effects, use in pregnancy, cost, etc.

Urinary tract infections in hospital are often caused by more resistant organisms than those in domiciliary practice and may be severe and require parenteral therapy. Cephalosporins are suitable agents for sensitive organisms and they achieve adequate serum and high urinary concentrations. They may be preferred to aminoglycosides in patients with renal impairment.

Intra-abdominal infections
Intra-abdominal infections are usually endogenous infections caused by organisms of the intestinal flora and consequently are frequently mixed, involving both aerobes and anaerobes. Treatment of such infections requires antibiotics active against both aerobes and anaerobes and this usually results in therapy with a combination of drugs, such as gentamicin and metronidazole or lincomycin. Most cephalosporins are unsuitable for use alone, as although the aerobic flora may be sensitive, *B. fragilis* strains are frequently resistant. However, cefoxitin and some of the newer cephalosporins show good activity against *B. fragilis* and it may be possible to replace combination therapy by treatment with cefoxitin or a single new cephalosporin. Studies with cefoxitin have shown promising results in this area but the lack of activity against *Ps. aeruginosa* makes this drug inadvisable for use in patients particularly susceptible to this organism, e.g. the immunosuppressed.

Biliary tract infections
The biliary tract presents a different picture because *B. fragilis* is an unusual pathogen in this site and infections are more commonly caused by enterobacteria, enterococci and occasionally *Cl. welchii*. When the infecting organism is sensitive, cephalosporins have been successful in the treatment of acute cholecystitis and related infections. Individual cephalosporins vary in the degree to which they are excreted in the bile (see this Chapter, under heading Pharmacology, Excretion) and the biliary excretion of some of the newer agents has not been studied in detail. Thus it is desirable to select the cephalosporin with optimum activity and biliary excretion. Cefazolin is favoured in this regard and

has also been used successfully as prophylaxis for biliary tract surgery[100]. Cephalosporins are not suitable for the treatment of *Str. faecalis*
infections since these organisms are resistant.

Septicaemia

In the clinical situation it is frequently necessary to commence treatment of a septicaemic patient before the infecting organism has been
isolated and its antibiotic sensitivity tested. An educated guess must be
made and a cephalosporin may be a reasonable choice, especially
cefoxitin with its activity against Gram-negative bacilli and anaerobes.
But in most instances a combination of gentamicin and metronidazole,
or a similar combination, is the first line of treatment. Further studies
are needed to define the use of cephalosporins in the treatment of
septicaemia.

Meningitis

The cephalosporins diffuse poorly into the cerebro-spinal fluid and
have been used relatively infrequently in the treatment of meningitis.
Cephaloridine has been reported to be successful in the treatment of
pneumococcal meningitis, but penicillin is preferable unless there are
strong contra-indications. Cefamandole has been used in the treatment
of *H. influenzae* meningitis caused by β-lactamase-producing strains
but the results are variable and chloramphenicol is preferable. There has
been a recent report that cefotaxime may have a useful role in the
treatment of bacterial meningitis[101].

Prophylaxis with cephalosporins

The cephalosporins have been widely used as prophylactic agents to
prevent infection arising from surgical or other invasive procedures in
patients. These occasions include peri-operative use in abdominal
surgery; peri- and post-operative use for implant surgery particularly
associated with joint prostheses; peri- and post-operative use in open-
heart surgery; pre-operatively in biliary surgery; and pre-operatively for
dental extraction in patients who are hypersensitive to penicillin.

CONCLUSIONS

The cephalosporin group of antibiotics contains compounds which may
differ markedly from other members of the group despite relatively
minor changes in chemical structure. These differences are seen not
only in antimicrobial activity both in degree and range, but also in
absorption, distribution and metabolic characteristics. The

differences in antimicrobial activity and in stability to β-lactamases produced by Gram-negative bacteria indicates that the various cephalosporins will have different clinical uses. Several important new compounds have recently become available for clinical use and the therapeutic position of these agents requires precise definition.

References

1 Newton, G. G. F. and Abraham, E. P. (1955). Cephalosporin, C, a new antibiotic containing sulphur and D-α-aminoadipic acid. *Nature*, **175**, 548

2 Brotzu, G. (1948). Lavori dell'istituto d'Igiene di Cagliari

3 Burton, H. S. and Abraham, E. P. (1951). Isolation of antibiotics from a species of *Cephalosporium*. Cephalosporins P_1, P_2, P_3, P_4 and P_5. *Biochem. J.*, **50**, 168

4 Crawford, K., Heatley, N. G., Boyd, P. F., Hale, C. W., Kelly, B. K., Miller, G. A. and Smith, N. (1952). Antibiotic production by a species of *Cephalosporium*. *J. Gen. Microbiol.*, **6**, 47

5 Abraham, E. P. and Newton, G. G. F. (1954). Synthesis of D-δ-amino-δ-carboxyvalerylglycine (a degradation product of cephalosporin N) and of DL-δ-amino-δ-carboxyvaleramide. *Biochem. J.*, **58**, 266

6 Godtfredsen, W. O., von Daehne, W. and van Gedal, S. (1965). The stereochemistry of fusidic acid. *Tetrahedron*, **21**, 3505

7 Florey, H. W. (1955). Antibiotic products of versatile fungus. *Ann. Int. Med.*, **43**, 480

8 Loder, P. B., Newton, G. G. F. and Abraham, E. P. (1961). The cephalosporin C nucleus (7-aminocephalosporanic acid) and some of its derivatives. *Biochem. J.*, **79**, 408

9 Strominger, J. L., Izaki, K., Matsuhashi, M. and Tipper, D. J. (1967). Peptidoglycan transpeptidase and D-alanine carboxypeptidase: penicillin-sensitive enzymatic reactions. *Proc. Fed. Am. Soc. Exp. Biol.*, **26**, 9

10 Tipper, D. J. and Strominger, J. L. (1965). Mechanism of action of penicillins: A proposal based on their structural similarity to acyl-D-alanyl-D-alanine. *Proc. Natl. Acad. Sci. USA*, **54**, 1133

11 O'Callaghan, C. H. and Muggleton, P. W. (1972). Biological reactions of cephalosporins and penicillins. In E. H. Flynn (ed.) *Cephalosporins and Penicillins*, p. 439. (New York and London: Academic Press)

12 Greenwood, D. and O'Grady, F. (1973). Comparison of the responses of *Escherichia coli* and *Proteus mirabilis* to seven beta-lactam antibiotics. *J. Infect. Dis.*, **128**, 211

13 Spratt, B. G. (1975). Distinct penicillin binding proteins involved in the division, elongation and shape of *Escherichia coli* K12. *Proc. Natl. Acad. Sci.*, **72**, 2999

14 Blumberg, P. M. and Strominger, J. L. (1974). Interaction of penicillin with the bacterial cell: penicillin-binding proteins and penicillin-sensitive enzymes. *Bacteriol. Rev.*, **38**, 291

15 Rolinson, G. N., MacDonald, A. C. and Wilson, D. A. (1977). Bactericidal action of beta-lactam antibiotics on *Escherichia coli* with particular reference to ampicillin and amoxycillin. *J. Antimicrob. Chemother.*, **3**, 541

16 Matthew, M. and Harris, A. M. (1976). Identification of beta-lactamases by analytical isoelectric focussing: correlation with bacterial taxonomy. *J. Gen. Microbiol.*, **94**, 55

17 Sykes, R. B. and Richmond, M. H. (1971). R factors, beta-lactamase and carbenicillin-resistant *Pseudomonas aeruginosa*. *Lancet*, **2**, 342

18 Hennessey, T. D. (1967). Inducible beta-lactamase in Enterobacter. *J. Gen. Microbiol.*, **49**, 277
19 Garber, N. and Friedman, J. (1970). Beta-lactamase and the resistance of *Pseudomonas aeruginosa* to various penicillins and cephalosporins. *J. Gen. Microbiol.*, **64**, 343
20 Sykes, R. B. and Matthew, M. (1976). The beta-lactamases of Gram-negative bacteria and their role in resistance to beta-lactam antibiotics. *J. Antimicrob. Chemother.*, **2**, 115
21 Matthew, M. (1979). Plasmid-mediated beta-lactamases of Gram-negative bacteria: properties and distribution. *J. Antimicrob. Chemother.*, **5**, Issue 4. (In press)
22 Medeiros, A. A. and O'Brien, T. F. (1975). Ampicillin-resistant *Haemophilus influenzae* type B possessing a TEM-type beta-lactamase but little permeability barrier to ampicillin. *Lancet*, **1**, 716
23 Aswapokee, N., Aswapokee, P., Fu, K. P. and Neu, H. C. (1978). *In vitro* activity and beta-lactamase stability of BL-S786 compared with those of other cephalosporins. *Antimicrob. Agents Chemother.*, **14**, 1
24 Johnson, V. L., Smith, I. M. and Habte-Gabr, E. (1978). Treatment with tobramycin and cefamandole, alone or together, in mice infected with *Escherichia coli* or *Staphylococcus aureus*. In: *Current Chemotherapy*. Proc. 10th International Congress of Chemotherapy, Vol. II, p. 789. (New York: American Society for Microbiology)
25 Brogden, R. N., Heel, R. C., Speight, T. M. and Avery, G. S. (1979). Cefoxitin: A review of its antibacterial activity, pharmacological properties and therapeutic use. *Drugs*, **17**, 1
26 Ernst, E. Chaim., Berger, S., Barza, M., Jacobus, N. V. and Tally, F. P. (1976). Activity of cefamandole and other cephalosporins against aerobic and anaerobic bacteria. *Antimicrob. Agents Chemother.*, **9**, 852
27 Wise, R., Rollason, T., Logan, M., Andrews, J. M. and Bedford, K. A. (1978). HR 756, a highly active cephalosporin: comparison with cefazolin and carbenicillin. *Antimicrob. Agents Chemother.*, **14**, 807
28 Sosna, J. P., Murray, P. R. and Medoff, G. (1978). Comparison of the *in vitro* activities of HR 756 with cephalothin, cefoxitin and cefamandole. *Antimicrob. Agents Chemother.*, **14**, 876
29 Shadomy, S., Wagner, G. and Carver, M. (1977). *In vitro* activities of five oral cephalosporins against aerobic pathogenic bacteria. *Antimicrob. Agents Chemother.*, **12**, 609
30 Bach, V. T., Khurana, M. M. and Thadepalli, H. (1978). *In vitro* activity of cefaclor against aerobic and anaerobic bacteria. *Antimicrob. Agents Chemother.*, **13**, 210
31 Kammer, R. B., Preston, D. A., Turner, J. R. and Hawley, L. C. (1975). Rapid detection of ampicillin-resistant *Haemophilus influenzae* and their susceptibility to sixteen antibiotics. *Antimicrob. Agents Chemother.*, **8**, 91
32 Drasar, W. A., Farrell, W., Howard, A. J., Hince, C., Leung, T. and Williams, J. D. (1978). Activity of HR 756 against *Haemophilus influenzae, Bacteroides fragilis* and Gram-negative rods. *J. Antimicrob. Chemother.*, **4**, 445
33 Williams, J. D. and Andrews, J. (1974). Sensitivity of *Haemophilus influenzae* to antibiotics. *Brit. Med. J.*, **1**, 134
34 Yourassowsky, E., Schoutens, E. and Vanderlinden, M. P. (1976). Antibacterial activity of eight cephalosporins against *Haemophilus influenzae* and *Streptococcus pneumoniae*. *J. Antimicrob. Chemother.*, **2**, 55
35 Sinai, R., Hammerberg, S., Marks, M. I. and Pai, C. H. (1978). *In vitro* suscep-

tibility of *Haemophilus influenzae* to sulfamethoxazole-trimethoprim and cefaclor, cephalexin and cephradine. *Antimicrob. Agents Chemother.*, **13**, 861

36 Strausbaugh, L. J., Mikhail, I. A. and Edman, D. C. (1978). Comparative *in vitro* activity of five cephalosporin antibiotics against Salmonellae. *Antimicrob. Agents Chemother.*, **13**, 134

37 Verbist, L. (1976). Comparison of the antibacterial activity of nine cephalosporins against *Enterobacteriaceae* and non-fermentative Gram-negative bacilli. *Antimicrob. Agents Chemother.*, **10**, 657

38 Chabbert, Y. A. and Lutz, A. J. (1978). HR 756, the *syn* isomer of a new methoxyimino cephalosporin with unusual antibacterial activity. *Antimicrob. Agents Chemother.*, **14**, 749

39 Chow, A. W. and Bednorz, D. (1978). Comparative *in vitro* activity of newer cephalosporins against anaerobic bacteria. *Antimicrob. Agents Chemother.*, **14**, 668

40 Vanhoof, R., Vanderlinden, M. P., Dierickx, R., Lauwers, S., Yourassowsky, E. and Butzler, J. P. (1978). Susceptibility of *Campylobacter fetus* subsp. *jejuni* to twenty-nine antimicrobial agents. *Antimicrob. Agents Chemother.*, **14**, 553

41 Goldstein, E. J. C., Sutter, V. L. and Finegold, S. M. (1978). Susceptibility of *Eikenella corrodens* to ten cephalosporins. *Antimicrob. Agents Chemother.*, **14**, 639

42 Appelbaum, P. C. and Chatterton, S. A. (1978). Susceptibility of anaerobic bacteria to ten antimicrobial agents. *Antimicrob. Agents Chemother.*, **14**, 371

43 Heymes, R., Lutz, A. and Schrinner, E. (1977). Experimental evaluation of HR 756, a new cephalosporin derivative. In *Current Chemotherapy*, Proc. 10th International Congress of Chemotherapy, Vol. II, p. 823. (New York: American Society for Microbiology)

44 Okonogi, K. Kida, M., Yoneda, M., Itoh, J. and Mitsuhashi, S. (1977). SCE-129, a new antipseudomonal cephalosporin and its biochemical properties. In *Current Chemotherapy*, Proc. 10th International Congress of Chemotherapy, Vol. II, p. 838. (New York: American Society for Microbiology)

45 Tosch, W., Kradolfer, F., Konopka, E. A., Regos, J., Zimmermann, W. and Zak, O. (1977). *In vitro* characterization of CGP 7174/E, a cephalosporin active against *Pseudomonas*. In *Current Chemotherapy*, Proc. 10th International Congress of Chemotherapy, Vol. II, p. 843. (New York: American Society for Microbiology)

46 Spyker, D. A., Thomas, B. L., Sande, M. A. and Bolton, W. K. (1978). Pharmacokinetics of cefaclor and cephalexin: dosage nomograms for impaired renal function. *Antimicrob. Agents Chemother.*, **14**, 172

47 Neiss, E. S. (1973). Cephradine – A summary of preclinical studies and clinical pharmacology. *J. Irish Med. Assoc.*, **66** (Suppl.), 1

48 Santoro, J., Agarwal, B. N., Martinelli, R., Wenger, N. and Levison, M. E. (1978). Pharmacology of cefaclor in normal volunteers and patients with renal failure. *Antimicrob. Agents Chemother.*, **13**, 951

49 Berman, S. J., Boughton, W. H., Sugihara, J. G., Wong, E. G. C., Sato, M. M. and Siemsen, A. W. (1978). Pharmacokinetics of cefaclor in patients with end stage renal disease and during haemodialysis. *Antimicrob. Agents Chemother.*, **14**, 281

50 Regamey, C. and Vonlanthen, M. (1977). Pharmacokinetics of cefamandole and cephalothin after intravenous administration in healthy adult volunteers and *in vitro* antibacterial spectrum. In *Current Chemotherapy*, Proc. 10th International Congress of Chemotherapy, Vol. II, p. 793. (New York: American Society for Microbiology)

51 Kucers, A. and Bennett, N.McK. (1975). *The Use of Antibiotics*. 2nd ed. (Heinemann)

cefazolin, cephalothin, and cephaloridine in the presence of biliary tract disease. *Antimicrob. Agents Chemother.*, **6**, 426

53 Naber, K. G. and Zinati, A. H. (1977). Pharmacokinetic studies and therapeutic evaluation of cefamandole in urology. In *Current Chemotherapy*, Proc. 10th International Congress of Chemotherapy, Vol. II, p. 801. (New York: American Society for Microbiology)

54 Daikos, G. K., Kosmidis, J. C., Stathakis, Ch. and Giamarellou, H. (1977). Cefuroxime: antimicrobial activity, human pharmacokinetics and therapeutic efficacy. *J. Antimicrob. Chemother.*, **3**, 555

55 Fitzgerald, R. H. Jr., Kelly, P. J., Snyder, R. J. and Washington, J. A. II. (1978). Penetration of methicillin, oxacillin and cephalothin into bone and synovial tissues. *Antimicrob. Agents Chemother.*, **14**, 723

56 Quinn, E. L., Madhavan, T., Wixson, R., Guise, E., Levin, N., Block, M., Burch, K., Fisher, E., Suarez, A. and del Busto, R. (1977). Cefamandole: observations on its spectrum, concentration in bone and bile, excretion in renal failure, and clinical efficacy. In *Current Chemotherapy*, Proc. 10th International Congress of Chemotherapy, Vol. II, p. 803. (New York: American Society for Microbiology)

57 Ellis, B. W., Stanbridge, R. de L., Sikorski, J. M., Dudley, H. A. F. and Spencer, R. C. (1975). Penetration into inflammatory exudate and wounds of two cephalosporins for the prevention of surgical infections. *J. Antimicrob. Chemother.*, **1**, 291

58 Gerding, D. N., Peterson, L. R., Legler, D. C., Hall, W. H. and Schierl, E. A. (1978). Ascitic fluid cephalosporin concentrations: influence of protein binding and serum pharmacokinetics. *Antimicrob. Agents Chemother.*, **14**, 234

59 Waterman, N. G. and Scharfenberger, L. F. (1978). Concentration relationships of cefaclor in serum, interstitial fluid, bile and urine of dogs. *Antimicrob. Agents Chemother.*, **14**, 614

60 Tschirkov, T., Eigel, P., Satter, P. and Knothe, H. (1977). Cefamandole and cephalothin in open-heart surgery: comparative pharmacokinetic appraisal. In *Current Chemotherapy*, Proc. 10th International Congress of Chemotherapy, Vol. II, p. 821. (New York: American Society for Microbiology)

61 Bergogne-Berezin, E., Kafe, H., Berthelot, G., Morel, C. and Benard, Y. (1977). Pharmacokinetic study of cefoxitin in bronchial secretions. In *Current Chemotherapy*, Proc. 10th International Congress of Chemotherapy, Vol. II, p. 758. (New York: American Society for Microbiology)

62 Axelrod, J. L. and Kochman, R. S. (1977). Cefamandole concentrations in human aqueous humor. In *Current Chemotherapy*, Proc. 10th International Congress of Chemotherapy, Vol. II, p. 799. (New York: American Society for Microbiology)

63 Vianna, N. J. and Kaye, D. (1967). Penetration of cephalothin into cerebro-spinal fluid. *Am. J. Med. Sci.*, **254**, 216

64 Oppenheimer, S., Beaty, H. N. and Petersdorf, R. G. (1969). Pathogenesis of meningitis. viii. Cerebro-spinal fluid and blood concentrations of methicillin, cephalothin, cephaloridine in experimental pneumococcal meningitis. *J. Lab. Clin. Med.*, **73**, 535

65 Brown, J. D., Mathies, A. W., Irler, D., Warren, W. S. and Leedom, J. M. (1969). Variable results of cephalothin therapy for meningococcal meningitis. In G. L. Hobby (ed.) *Antimicrobial Agents and Chemotherapy*, p. 432. (New York: American Society for Microbiology)

66 Editorial. (1973). Antibiotic-induced meningitis. *Brit. Med. J.*, **3**, 366

67 Ruedy, J. (1967). The concentration of cephaloridine in cerebrospinal fluid of rabbits with experimental meningitis. *Postgrad. Med. J.*, **43**, (Suppl.), 146

68 Lerner, P. I. (1971). The penetration of cephaloridine into cerebrospinal fluid. *Am. J. Med. Sci.*, **262**, 321

69 Walker, S. H. and Gahol, V. P. (1978). Pharmacokinetics of cefamandole in infants and children. *Antimicrob. Agents Chemother.*, **14**, 315

70 Liu, C., Baker, L. H., Gerjarusak, P., Romig, D. A., Hinthorn, D. R., Smith, H. and Harris, J. L. (1975). Penetration of cefazolin and cefamandole into cerebrospinal fluid. In 9th International Congress of Chemotherapy Abstract no. M-223

71 Hinthorn, D. R., Liu, C., Hodges, G. R., Dworzack, D. L., Rosett, W. and Harms, J. (1977). Cerebrospinal fluid penetration of cefoxitin and experience in treatment of bacterial infections. In *Current Chemotherapy*, Proc. 10th International Congress of Chemotherapy, Vol. II, p. 757. (New York: American Society for Microbiology)

72 Brogard, J. M., Haegele, P., Dorner, M. and Lavillaureux, J. (1973). Biliary excretion of a new semisynthetic cephalosporin, cephacetrile. *Antimicrob. Agents Chemother.*, **3**, 19

73 Ram, M. D. and Watanatittan, S. (1973). Levels of cefazolin in human bile. *J. Infect. Dis.* (Suppl.), **128**, 361

74 Nishida, M., Murakawa, T., Matsubara, T., Kohno, Y., Yokota, Y., Yasutomi, T. and Okamoto, M. (1976). Characteristics of biliary excretion of cefazolin and other cephalosporins with reference to the relationship between serum levels and administration conditions. *Chemotherapy*, **22**, 30

75 Sales, J. E. L., Sutcliffe, M. B. and O'Grady, F. (1969). Cephalexin and the biliary tract. In R. O. Foord (ed.) *Proc. Symp. Clinical Evaluation of Cephalexin*, p. 42. (London: Royal Society of Medicine)

76 Levine, B. B. (1973). Antigenicity and cross-reactivity of penicillins and cephalosporins. *J. Infect. Dis.* **128** (Suppl.), S 364

77 Dewdney, J. M. and Weston, B. (1976). Immune responsiveness to β-lactam antibiotics. In *Proc. 9th International Congress of Chemotherapy*, Vol. 4, p. 261. (Plenum Press)

78 Levine, B. B., Redmond, A. P., Fellner, M. J. *et al.* (1966). Penicillin allergy and the heterogenous immune responses of man to benzyl penicillin. *J. Clin. Invest.*, **45**, 1895

79 Dash, C. H. (1975). Penicillin allergy and the cephalosporins. *J. Antimicrob. Chemother.*, **1** (Suppl.), 107

80 Levine, B. B. and Zolov, D. M. (1969). Prediction of penicillin allergy by immunological tests. *J. Allergy*, **43**, 231

81 Thoburn, R., Johnson, J. E. and Cluff, L. E. (1966). Studies on the epidemiology of adverse drug reactions. IV. The relationship of cephalothin and penicillin allergy. *J. Am. Med. Assoc.*, **198**, 345

82 Sanders, W. E. Jr., Johnson, J. E. and Taggart, J. G. (1974). Adverse reactions to cephalothin and cephapirin. *New Engl. J. Med.*, **290**, 424

83 Foord, R. D. (1975). Cephaloridine, cephalothin and the kidney. *J. Antimicrob. Chemother.*, **1** (Suppl.), 119

84 Tune, B. M. and Kempson, R. L. (1973). Nephrotoxic drugs (corres.), *Brit. Med. J.*, **3**, 635

85 Linsell, W. D., Pines, A. and Hayden, J. W. (1967). Hyaline cast formation in patients treated with cephaloridine. *J. Clin. Pathol.*, **20**, 857

86 Fillastre, J. P., Laumonier, R., Humbert, G., Dubois, D., Metayer, J., Delpech, A., LeRoy, J. and Robert, M. (1973). Acute renal failure associated with combined gentamicin and cephalothin therapy. *Brit. Med. J.*, **2**, 396

87 Kleinknecht, D., Ganeval, D. and Dioz, D. (1973). Acute renal failure after high

doses of gentamicin and cephalothin. *Lancet*, **1**, 1129

88 Wade, J. C., Petty, B. G., Conrad, G., Smith, C. R., Lipsky, J. J., Ellner, J. and Lietman, P. S. (1978). Cephalothin plus an aminoglycoside is more nephrotoxic than methicillin plus an aminoglycoside. *Lancet*, **2**, 604

89 Harrison, W. O., Silverblatt, F. J. and Turck, M. (1975). Gentamicin nephrotoxicity; failure of three cephalosporins to potentiate injury in rats. *Antimicrob. Agents Chemother.*, **8**, 209

90 Dellinger, P., Murphy, T., Pinn, V., Barza, M. and Weinstein, L. (1976). Protective effect of cephalothin against gentamicin-induced nephrotoxicity in rats. *Antimicrob. Agents Chemother.*, **10**, 80

91 Welles, J. S. (1972). Pharmacology and toxicology of cephalosporins. In E. H. Flynn (ed.) *Cephalosporins and Penicillins, Chemistry and Biology*, p. 583. (New York: Academic Press)

92 Silverblatt, F., Harrison, W. O. and Turck, M. (1973). Nephrotoxicity of cephalosporin antibiotics in experimental animals. *J. Infect. Dis.*, **128** (Suppl.), S 367

93 Wold, J. S., Welles, J. S., Owen, N. V., Gibson, W. R. and Morton, D. M. (1978). Toxicologic evaluation of cefamandole nafate in laboratory animals. *J. Infect. Dis.*, **137** (Suppl.), 51

94 Capel-Edwards, K., Atkinson, R. M., Pratt, D. A. H. and Patterson, G. G. (1977). The toxicology of cefuroxime. *Proc. R. Soc. Med.*, **70** (Suppl. 9), 11

95 Trollfors, B., Norrby, R. and Kristianson, K. (1977). Effect on renal function of treatment with cefoxitin alone or in combination with furosemide. In *Current Chemotherapy*, Proc. 10th International Congress of Chemotherapy, Vol. II, p. 760. (New York: American Society for Microbiology)

96 Murdoch, J. (1964). Clinical trial of cephaloridine. *Brit. Med. J.*, **2**, 1238

97 Stewart, G. T. and Holt, R. J. (1964). Laboratory and clinical results with cephaloridine. *Lancet*, **2**, 1305

98 Martin, W. J. and Wellmann, W. E. (1967). Clinically useful antimicrobial agents. *Postgrad. Med. J. (Suppl.)*, **43**, 142

99 Gralnick, H. R., McGinniss, M. and Halterman, R. (1972). Thrombocytopenia with sodium cephalothin therapy. *Ann. Intern. Med.*, **77**, 401

100 Wise, R., Stachan, C. J. L. and Powis, S. J. A. (1977). Cefazolin in biliary surgery. In *Current Chemotherapy*, Proc. 10th International Congress of Chemotherapy, Vol. II, p. 854. (New York: American Society for Microbiology)

101 Brown, W. M. and Fallon, R. J. (1979). Cefotaxime for bacterial meningitis. *Lancet*, **1**, 1246

4

Anaerobic infections and their treatment

R. Wise and M. N. Logan

INTRODUCTION

History

The scientific study of anaerobic bacteria began with the observations of Louis Pasteur in 1861, although a century earlier an Italian priest, Lazaro Spallanzani, had observed anaerobic organisms but failed to appreciate their significance. Pasteur recorded that 'the ferment which produces butyric acid is an infusorium living in the complete absence of oxygen'[1]. In these investigations he observed rod-shaped bacteria killed in the presence of oxygen. In 1878 Pasteur reported with Joubert and Chamberland a strictly anaerobic 'Sepsis Vibrio'[2].

Clinical tetanus was described by Hippocrates (460–355 BC). In 1889 Kitasato[3] cultured tetanus bacilli in an atmosphere of hydrogen, and in 1890 Behring and Kitasato discovered tetanus anti-toxin. Two years later Nuttall and Welch discovered an anaerobic spore-bearing organism causing gas gangrene (*Clostridium welchii*, later known as *Cl. perfringens*). In 1898 Veillon isolated Gram-negative non-sporing anaerobes from various lesions in 25 cases of foetid and gangrenous suppuration. The same year Hallé isolated similar organisms from cases of otitis media and from the blood of 18 patients from suppurative conditions associated with jaundice, all of whom died.

The 1914–18 war stimulated energetic research into the treatment of wound sepsis, gas gangrene and tetanus. Difficulty in culturing *Cl. perfringens* led to the invention of the McIntosh and Fildes anaerobic jar, still in use. The 1939–45 war produced further refinements with the development of a liquid medium for the growth of anaerobic bacteria. Alongside development in understanding and diagnosis, advances were being made in treatment and prophylaxis of gas gangrene. Acridine dyes were introduced into wound therapy in World War I but later fell into disuse. The 'thirties saw the advent of sulphonamides and anti-toxins. During the Second World War the case fatality from gas gangrene fell steadily from 50% to 22%. This was related to earlier and more effective surgery, the introduction and intensive use of chemotherapeutic and serological agents and advances in transfusion and resuscitation techniques. Florey and Cairns first reported the use of penicillin in gas gangrene in 1943[4].

Tetanus was another great scourge of war and during the early years of World War I, 8 of every 1000 wounded British soldiers died of tetanus. In 1920 Clenny and Ramon discovered independently that tetanus toxoid could be made by treating the toxin with formaldehyde. The prophylactic use of the toxoid led to an impressive fall in the incidence of tetanus among the wounded of World War II.

Although recognised as a human pathogen by Veillon and Zuber in 1898, the last decade has seen a surge of interest and recognition of the *Bacteroides* group as an important cause of anaerobic sepsis. There have been sporadic references to the pathogenicity of this organism throughout this century. Alston[5] in a review article reports isolates of *Bacteroides* in 12 patients in a hospital in North London between 1933 and 1944. Between 1944 and 1965 he reported no further isolates even though these were specifically searched for. During the nineteen fifties cases of severe infection due to *Bacteroides* were reported by MacLennan[6], Gillespie and Guy[7] and Gunn[8], following gastrointestinal surgery particularly in the elderly and following surgery for carcinoma and gynaecological conditions. *Bacteroides* had also been implicated in oropharyngeal sepsis and abscesses of the lung and brain.

Concurrent with the more general recognition as a pathogen that the *Bacteroides* now enjoy, have been advances in suitable chemotherapy. Prior to the introduction of sulphonamides the mortality of infections with *Bacteroides* was 81%. The use of sulphonamides alone led to a reduction to 64% and combination with penicillin and streptomycin to 50%. Gunn (1956)[8] reports sensitivity of *Bacteroides* to erythromycin and chloramphenicol and suggests that such broad spectrum antibiotics should be used.

Within the last few years considerable advances have been made in understanding the treatment of anaerobic infections. In this brief review we shall try and cover the most important diseases and also examine the antibiotics used.

Laboratory aspects of diagnosis
Anaerobic bacteria fall into one of several groups according to their

intolerance to oxygen. This has clinical and laboratory importance. The highly oxygen intolerant bacteria which make up part of the normal body flora are extremely difficult to grow and probably of little clinical importance. The majority of strains met in clinical practice show variable oxygen tolerance and anaerobes can be defined as bacteria which are unable to initiate growth unless the oxidation–reduction potential of the environment is low. Other bacteria prefer to grow in a reduced oxygen environment, yet will tolerate some oxygen – the microaerophilic bacteria. Facultative anaerobes include the majority of pathogens such as *Escherichia coli* and *Staphylococcus aureus,* which will grow aerobically or anaerobically.

It has been found that the enzyme superoxide dismutase, which is present in aerobic bacteria, is absent in anaerobes[54]. This enzyme converts the toxic O_2^- radical to H_2O_2. The absence of the enzyme would lead to accumulation of this toxin.

It is important for the clinician to have some knowledge of these facts as it is obvious that bacteria which are sensitive to air will only be recovered from correct specimens suitably transported. The best type of specimen is pus itself, sent in a sealed universal container or in a plugged syringe or, failing this, a well taken swab rapidly transported to the laboratory. If any specimen is delayed unduly in reaching the laboratory, the likelihood of recovering anaerobes from that specimen is diminished. Certain centres[9] with a particular interest in anaerobic diseases may take care of their specimens using such means as 'gassed out' tubes etc.

There is little point in sending specimens to the bacteriology laboratory for anaerobic examination if the specimen is contaminated with anaerobes. Almost pure faeces discharging from a wound is an all too common example of an unnecessary specimen which will yield no useful information. Expectorated sputum will always yield anaerobes – from the oral flora present in the contaminating saliva – so that a transtracheal aspirate is needed. Attempting to diagnose an intra-uterine infection from a high vaginal swab is likewise fraught with problems of contamination from the vaginal flora.

As with all serious infections at whatever site, blood cultures should be taken. This is particularly important as *Bacteroides fragilis* is a common isolate from blood cultures taken in those centres which have a special interest in anaerobic bacteriology. The lower isolation rate from other centres probably reflects reduced clinical awareness just as much as less efficient laboratory techniques.

It is not the purpose of this review to cover the problems of laboratory diagnosis, but the clinician should realise that the diagnosis of anaerobic infection may be a little slower than with aerobic infection. It will probably take two days for the anaerobic organisms to grow and then maybe a further two days before the sensitivity of the pathogen has been determined. More rapid methods are being developed. The injection of a simple extract of pus into a gas-liquid chromatography column may well give a tracing indicative of certain volatile fatty acids which are produced in the pus by these organisms. An example is shown in Figure 1, and in this case we were able to report to the surgeon that he was probably dealing with an anaerobic infection within 45 minutes of receiving the specimen. The clinician may recognise the common putrid smell. This is characteristic of anaerobic infections. A brick red fluorescence of pus, or pus soaked material, under ultra-violet light is characteristic of *Bacteroides melaninogenicus*. A simple and rapid test is a Gram stain which, when examined by an experienced technician, may well increase suspicion of an anaerobic infection.

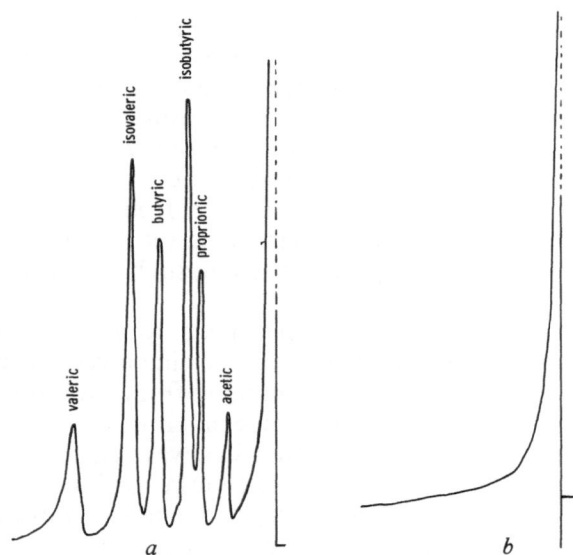

Figure 1 (a) Gas liquid chromatography tracing of pus from which was cultured *B. fragilis*. (b) Gas liquid chromatography tracing of pus from which was cultured *S aureus*

Anaerobic bacteria and their classifications

The majority of bacteria present in man are anaerobes. They are broadly classified by shape and Gram staining reaction.

Of the Gram-positive rods (or bacilli) *Clostridium perfringens* (*Cl. welchii*) is common in the intestinal tract of man and animals. They form hardy spores and like *Cl. tetani* can exist for long periods in soil. The diseases caused are closely related to the exotoxins produced.

The skin of man is colonised by other Gram-positive rods – the proprionibacteria and, in the mouth, *Actinomyces.* Bifidobacteria are widely found in the mouth, gut and vagina.

Gram-negative rods, in particular the *Bacteroides* group have, as has been stated, only relatively recently assumed importance clinically. The subdivisions of this group are complex and the finer points of little relevance to the practising clinician. The most important is *B. fragilis* which is part of the normal flora of the gut and vagina. *B. oralis* is found in the mouth and nasopharynx and *B. melaninogenicus* can be found in mouth, vagina and gut. Other Gram-negative bacilli, such as *Fusobacterium,* are widely distributed in the body.

The anaerobic cocci are also found in the mouth, vagina and gut and of these the anaerobic streptococcus is the most important. Anaerobic spirochaetes can also cause problems – the best known being *Borrelia vincentii* and its association with gingivitis ('trench mouth').

In most sites of the body the aerobes are outnumbered by the anaerobes[10] by a factor of up to 100 000. It is not surprising, therefore, that they are implicated in many bacterial diseases. They may also be important in the pathogenesis of other diseases, even cancer[11] and in a lighter vein it has been said that every smell emanating from the human body is due to anaerobes.

DISEASES CAUSED BY ANAEROBES AND THEIR TREATMENT

General considerations
More often than not, when the clinician receives the bacteriology laboratory report of a specimen from which he expects to grow anaerobes, it will describe a mixed bacterial population, usually an aerobe together with an anaerobe. In one series of 67 cases of abdominal sepsis studied by Finegold *et al.*[12], 193 bacterial anaerobic isolates were found and 129 aerobes. In that study, therefore, an average of 4–5 different species were isolated in each patient. Most routine bacteriology laboratories do not go to such lengths of indentification, but this does emphasise that anaerobic infections are rarely purely anaerobic in nature and are, more often than not, multi-pathogenic.

It is interesting to speculate on why many anaerobic infections also have aerobes present. One of the traditional views is that the aerobes can remove or reduce the amount of oxygen present so allowing the anaerobes to grow. For example tetanus spores will not germinate in laboratory animals unless facultative bacteria are present[13]. On the other hand, in Meleney's 'synergistic gangrene' it appears that a *Staph. aureus* produces a hyaluronidase which will then permit the microaerophilic streptococcus to spread in the tissues[14]. Yet another example of aerobe/anaerobe interaction is in necrotic anaerobic processes involving mucous membrane, in which a diphtheroid appears to produce vitamin K – a requirement for *B. melaninogenicus*[15].

Many anaerobic infections are pus forming and some studies have shown interesting interactions between the environment and the bacteria. Polymorphs function less efficiently at phagocytosis under the anaerobic environment of such an abscess. Also inhibition of phagocytosis by certain anaerobic bacteria *in vitro* has been described[16]. It has been postulated that the anaerobes are protecting the aerobes.

Infections caused by anaerobes fall into two main groups. The toxin mediated diseases of the clostridia, namely botulism and tetanus, will not be discussed here. Rather we will discuss the septic infections about which our understanding has increased considerably in the last few years.

As in the treatment of any bacterial disease, antimicrobial agents are only one facet of treatment. This is especially true in anaerobic infections where it is often necessary to approach the management of the patient from several directions. As has been said, anaerobes are often pus-forming, and surgical drainage is all important when an abscess is present. This will remove the majority of organisms, improve the oxygenation of the tissues and limit toxin formation. In some anaerobic infections it may be necessary to use hyperbaric oxygen as a means of increasing tissue oxygen perfusion. The use of specific anti-toxins in clostridial infections may also have a part to play.

There are a fairly small number of antimicrobials which are of importance in the treatment of anaerobic infections, and these will be discussed briefly. Table 1 summarises the antibacterial activity of the agents against the more common anaerobes.

The available antibiotics

Penicillins
The penicillin group of antibiotics (which include ampicillin and carbenicillin) are active against a wide range of anaerobes but the commonest pathogen, *B. fragilis,* is resistant to all but high levels of these drugs. This is because *B. fragilis* in common with many pathogens, such as many strains of *E. coli* and *Staph. aureus,* produces enzymes (β-lactamases) which destroy penicillins[17]. There is now direct evidence to show that such degradation does occur *in vivo*[18]. Some success in the treatment of anaerobic infections with carbenicillin has

Table 1 Sensitivity of common anaerobes to antimicrobial agents

	Penicillin G	Lincomycin/ Clindamycin	Metronidazole	Chloramphenicol	Tetracycline	Erythromycin	Cefoxitin
B. fragilis	+	+++	++++	+++	++	++	++
Bacteroides spp. (inc. *B. melaninogenicus* and *oralis*)	++	+++	++++	+++	++	++	++
Fusobacterium spp.	++++	+++	++++	+++	+++	+	+++
Anaerobic cocci	+++	++++	+++[1]	+++	++	++	+++
Clostridium spp.	++++	+++	++++	+++	++	+	++

1 Microaerophilic strains (not true anaerobes) are resistant
+ Strains usually resistant – should not be used
++ Strains often resistant – should not be used
+++ Most strains sensitive – may be used
++++ Almost all strains sensitive – good choice

Table 2 The combination of penicillin and clavulanic acid against *B. fragilis*. Minimum inhibitory concentration of benzylpenicillin (μg/ml) when present with three concentrations of clavulanic acid[†]

Strain no.	Penicillin alone	Penicillin + 10 μg/ml clavulanic acid	Penicillin + 5 μg/ml clavulanic acid	Penicillin + 1 μg/ml clavulanic acid
1	8	< 0.01	2	1
2	8	< 0.01	4	8
3	16	< 0.01	0.5	0.5
4	512	< 0.01	4	4
5	256	< 0.01	0.12	1

† From Tally *et al.* (1978)[23]

been reported[19]. This is possibly related to the very large doses of this drug which are usually employed, so that the amount of antibiotic overcomes the effect of the β-lactamase. An interesting development in penicillin therapy is the appearance of a compound, clavulanic acid, which structurally resembles the β-lactam drugs yet has little or no antimicrobial activity. Clavulanic acid is, however, a potent inhibitor of β-lactamases[20] and when combined with benzylpenicillin it potentiates the latter's activity considerably[21] (Table 2). Some of the newer penicillins such as mezlocillin and piperacillin have an enhanced degree of activity against *B. fragilis* and results of clinical trials with these compounds are awaited with interest.

Benzylpenicillin is active against many anaerobic species other than *B. fragilis,* although some strains may be rather resistant. For the treatment of chest infections where mixed organisms are the rule, large doses of penicillin may be satisfactory. As an adjuvant to the surgical treatment of gas gangrene, benzylpenicillin should be administered; all strains of *Clostridium perfringens* are sensitive, but certain other clostridia may be highly resistant. Some strains of anaerobic cocci show moderate resistance and reports of resistance in *B. melaninogenicus* are appearing. If benzylpenicillin is to be used, it should be administered in large doses, possibly in excess of 20 mega units per day. Even at this dose it is a safe drug but to achieve comparable levels with such agents as ampicillin or amoxycillin one would have to use doses which would be accompanied by an unacceptable incidence of side effects. The usefulness of these two agents in the treatment of anaerobic infections is therefore very doubtful.

Lincomycin and clindamycin
Lincomycin and its 7-chloro derivative, clindamycin, are of considerable use in the treatment of anaerobic infections. Clindamycin, being more active than lincomycin, is the preferred agent. The vast majority of anaerobic Gram-negative rods are sensitive but a significant number of strains of clostridia show resistance. Clindamycin can be given orally or by injection and has been used in the treatment of a very wide range of anaerobic infections: its efficacy alone and when used in combination with other agents such as the aminoglycosides has been proved.

The use of many antibiotics, but in particular clindamycin and lincomycin, has been implicated in the aetiology of pseudomembranous colitis. This occurs rarely, fortunately, and it can be fatal. The aetiology is only just becoming understood. It appears that a clostridium (*Cl. difficile*) for some reason, possibly being resistant to the antibiotic in question, increases in number and elaborates a toxin which causes the bowel injury[22]. This problem should not detract from the great usefulness of clindamycin in anaerobic infections but rather should caution the clinician about its use in the treatment of trivial infections. Another important reason why these antibiotics should be used with care is that there is now evidence that clindamycin resistance can be transferred from one *B. fragilis* to another by means of a plasmid (R factor)[23].

Metronidazole

This agent was originally introduced for the treatment of vaginitis caused by *Trichomonas vaginalis*. It was the clever observation of a British dental surgeon that a patient with Vincent's gingivitis improved on this agent and subsequently its benefit in the treatment of a wide range of anaerobic infections has been well documented. The drug has also been used extensively in the prophylaxis of anaerobic infections following abdominal and gynaecological operations. Almost all anaerobes are inhibited by this agent. Certain streptococci, which are probably microaerophilic rather than true anaerobes, are resistant. Aerobic organisms are not inhibited by this compound. One exception is the causative organism of an increasingly recognised form of enteritis due to a campylobacter (*C. jejuni*) which is inhibited.

Metronidazole can be used by the oral, parenteral or per-rectal route and it appears to cross the blood–brain barrier well.

The usual dose employed in the treatment of anaerobic infections is 400 mg three times a day by mouth or a 1 g suppository 8-hourly.

Other drugs of the nitroimidazole family are tinidazole and nimorazole. The activities are similar but there are differences in pharmacology.

With the large and recent increase in usage of metronidazole it is salutary to note yet again that the overenthusiastic use of an antibiotic is often quickly followed by the appearance of bacterial resistance. Reports of strains of *B. fragilis* insusceptible to metronidazole are now appearing[24] [25]. This seems to be associated with long term therapy. The message is clear – important antimicrobials such as metronidazole should be reserved for clearly defined indications and the length of therapy should not exceed 7–10 days.

Chloramphenicol

This antimicrobial has a high degree of activity against anaerobic bacteria and resistance is rare. The haematological adverse reactions are well known but this should not deter the clinician from using this drug when it is indicated. Chloramphenicol is an amphoteric molecule of high lipid solubility. It can, therefore, penetrate all body tissues to a greater extent than many other antimicrobials. Finegold[26] considers that chloramphenicol is the drug of choice in treatment of serious anaerobic infections, particularly of the central nervous system, where the organism or its drug sensitivity are unknown. More recently some doubt on the efficacy of chloramphenicol has emerged. It has been shown[27] that in a rat intra-abdominal abscess, clostridia and *B. fragilis* can inactivate chloramphenicol, which may explain the failure of the drug in certain instances of severe anaerobic infections. The usual dose is 500 mg four times daily.

Erythromycin
Although this antibiotic is at times very useful and safe its role in the treatment of anaerobic infections is limited. It is very active against Gram-positive anaerobes (such as anaerobic cocci and *Cl. perfringens*) and *B. melaninogenicus*. It cannot be considered as having any reliable activity against *B. fragilis*. It has been suggested[28] that this *in vitro* resistance may be due more to methodological problems rather than representing true resistance and there have been reports (often difficult to interpret) of treating so-called resistant organisms with erythromycin, with good results. As there are other, potentially more reliable agents available for use we think that erythromycin should not be used in the treatment of anaerobic sepsis unless the organism is known to be sensitive.

Tetracyclines
Although once widely used in the treatment of anaerobic infections, tetracyclines have fallen from favour. This is due in part to the emergence of resistance of *B. fragilis* to this group of drugs. About one quarter of all *B. fragilis* are resistant. Resistance in *Cl. perfringens* has also been noted. Again the development of metronidazole and clindamycin, which are more predictable in their activity, must have contributed to the decline in use of this agent. Two newer derivatives, doxycycline and minocycline are more active than tetracycline, and some tetracycline resistant strains are susceptible to these two agents. Both have been shown to be clinically effective.

Cephalosporins/cephamycins
The cephalosporins, by and large, have a good degree of activity against many anaerobes, in particular the anaerobic cocci and *Clostridium* spp. They, like many agents, are inadequate in their activity against *B. fragilis* (Table 3). The new agent cefoxitin which is a cephamycin (a molecular addition to the cephalosporin ring) does have a useful degree of activity against most aerobes and anaerobes. This implies that

Table 3 The activity of 6 cephalosporin antibiotics against 20 strains of *Bacteroides fragilis*†

	Minimum inhibitory concentration (μg/ml)							
	1	2	4	8	16	32	64	>64
Cefoxitin		5	7	4	3	1		
Cephalothin				3	3	4		10
Cephaloridine		3	1	5			6	5
Cefuroxime			13	2			1	4
Cephazolin			2	12	2			4
Cephalexin				4	9	3		4

† Authors' unpublished observations

cefoxitin may well have a role to play in the treatment of infections where mixed aerobes and anaerobes are implicated, as is often the case in abdominal sepsis. First clinical reports are encouraging[29]. The usual dose is 1–2 g i.v. every 6–8 h although in severely ill cases up to 5 g, 8-hourly have been used.

Other agents
It should be remembered that the aminoglycosides (gentamicin, kanamycin, tobramycin, streptomycin and amikacin) have no useful activity against anaerobes, and when they are being used in the treatment of serious undiagnosed sepsis, in which an anaerobe could be implicated, they should be combined with one of the other agents listed above.

There is conflicting *in vitro* and clinical information on the activity of co-trimoxazole and its use for anaerobic infections is probably best avoided. More recently[30] there has been some interest in the combination of trimethoprim with rifampicin, which shows synergistic activity against *B. fragilis*, but no clinical information is available.

Spectinomycin, an antibiotic usually reserved for the treatment of gonorrhoea, has some modest activity against *B. fragilis* but this is unlikely to be of much clinical significance[31].

Treatment of specific infections

Chest infections
The respiratory tract below the epiglottis is normally sterile. The common aerobic pathogens, such as pneumococci and *H. influenzae* are

normal upper respiratory tract commensals in a proportion of people. Concomitant viral illness or structural abnormalities probably are common reasons for colonisation of the lower respiratory tract by these aerobes. In the case of anaerobic infections the anaerobes isolated most probably also originated from the oro-pharynx. Aspiration of oropharyngeal secretions is the most important cause of anaerobic chest infections. The area of lung involved will be determined by the position of the patient at the time of aspiration. In over one half of such infections anaerobes are the only organisms present, and often there is more than one anaerobe per case. In one series from the United States[32] the commonest bacterial isolates were anaerobic streptococci, *B. melaninogenicus* and *Fusobacterium* spp. Interestingly *B. fragilis* was also quite common (although this is not a normal commensal of the upper respiratory tract). The majority of information on anaerobic chest infections comes from the United States, where they appear to be more common. More importantly, there is a greater sense of awareness of anaerobic infections there, possibly better laboratory facilities (in some centres) but also, and more significantly, far better specimen collection by transtracheal aspiration.

Anaerobic chest infections include a variety of aetiologically linked conditions such as lung abscess, aspiration pneumonia and empyema. Where pus has formed it would be advisable to drain this if possible – by physiotheraphy, bronchoscopy or surgical intervention. Antibiotics should also be given, and it is of considerable interest to note that benzylpenicillin is just as efficacious as the more recently introduced clindamycin. In one study Finegold *et al.*[33] showed that, in spite of the fact that *B. fragilis* was not uncommon in such infections (and resistant to penicillin), patients responded equally well to either drug. This suggests that the isolation of *B. fragilis* in pulmonary infections does not necessarily mean that therapy should be altered from benzylpenicillin.

The length of treatment will be dictated by the condition, and in cases of lung abscess this may be as long as 12 weeks. In the more acute aspiration pneumonia, therapy should continue until the patient responds, and the temperature and pulse fall, and then be continued for about one week. X-ray improvement usually takes much longer and may be a poor guide. It should be remembered that aerobes may also be present in these infections and often therapy will have to be tailored to the individual by using a combination of antibiotics.

Central nervous system infections
Anaerobes are common pathogens of the central nervous system, usually causing intracranial abscesses rather than pyogenic meningitis. The abscess appears to develop by contiguous spread from infections in

such sites as the middle ear and paranasal sinuses. Less commonly, spread is metastatic from infections elsewhere – usually in the lungs, such as bronchiectasis or lung abscess. It is interesting to speculate on how these organisms travel from lung to brain tissue. It has been postulated that the valve-free spinal venous system is the route and this is assisted by an increased intrathoracic pressure as occurs in coughing. It has been suggested that previous cerebrovascular accidents may predispose to brain abscess formation[34].

The commonest site for brain abscesses is in the temporal lobe (the commonest underlying condition being chronic otitis media) and the most frequent pathogens are *Bacteroides* spp. (usually the more resistant *B. fragilis*). Anaerobic streptococci and *Fusobacterium* spp. are also frequently isolated. Again the anaerobes are often in mixed culture, with other anaerobes and with facultative bacteria.

The diagnosis of intracranial abscess has improved recently with the addition of computer assisted tomography to the other procedures, such as arteriography, radioisotope scanning and EEG. Except in very early cases it is usually impossible to avoid surgery, which may involve repeated aspiration or excision. Surgery should be accompanied by intensive antimicrobial therapy. Most antibiotics penetrate poorly into the CSF unless the meninges are inflamed. Similarly penetration into the highly lipid tissues of the brain is also poor. To get reasonable levels of penicillin in pus from patients with intracranial abscess large doses (over 10 g/day) have to be given[35]. Two antibiotics which are lipophilic and attain satisfactory concentrations in such pus are chloramphenicol and metronidazole[36], both of which appear to be concentrated at this site. In a recent review of the subject[37] it is recommended that abscesses of the frontal lobe (often originating from infections in the sinuses), if caused by penicillin-sensitive streptococci, be treated with penicillin (in large doses). Those of otitic origin in the temporal lobe, often yielding a mixed flora, demand multiple chemotherapy – possibly chloramphenicol and metronidazole with maybe penicillin or co-trimoxazole in addition. Spinal abscesses are usually staphylococcal, and fusidic acid is the drug of choice. It would seem reasonable to use one of these agents either alone, if the organism is known, but if not then in combination with other agents.

Urinary tract infections

The recovery of anaerobic organisms from urine is low and this is presumably related to the fact that although urine is an excellent cultural environment for most facultative bacteria it is very poor for anaerobes as the partial pressure of oxygen is too high. One group of workers[38] examined 15 250 samples of voided urine and found significant numbers of anaerobes in only 1% and in no case was the anaerobe thought to be of clinical importance. Finegold[32] has reviewed the documented cases of anaerobic infections of the urinary tract. Simple cystitis is rare but anaerobes have been isolated from renal and perinephric abscesses, infections of the periurethral tissues and prostate and from pyelonephritis. In cystitis when an anaerobe has been isolated it is often accompanied by a more readily recognised pathogen, such as *E. coli*. The commonest anaerobes were anaerobic cocci, *Bacteroides* spp. and *Clostridium* spp.

Clinicians should, therefore, view with suspicion a laboratory report of an anaerobe from a urine specimen. They should be advised to repeat the investigation and then, if positive, consider the possibility of other concomitant pathology of the urinary tract.

Intra-abdominal infections

It has already been mentioned that the flora of the intestinal tract of man is predominantly anaerobic. This is certainly true distal to the lower ileum, when the numbers of anaerobes vastly outnumber the aerobes. This is in contrast to the stomach and proximal small bowel, where the flora reflects the bacteria in swallowed saliva, aerobes predominating, and the numbers of anaerobes far smaller. Sepsis related to perforations of the gastrointestinal tract will, therefore, reflect this difference in flora. Sepsis and morbidity is less with gastric or duodenal perforation, than with injuries to the colon. Intra-abdominal infection is therefore usually related to spillage of large bowel contents. This also means that such infections are almost always polymicrobial. In one large study[39] anaerobes were isolated from 84% of patients with intra-abdominal infections and aerobes only in 36%. These workers also found an average of four organisms per case. *B. fragilis* as would be expected accounts for about one third of all the anaerobes isolated in that study, but Gorbach *et al.*[40] found *B. fragilis* accounted for 65% of anaerobic isolates.

Intra-abdominal infections whether caused by rupture of a viscus, as in acute appendicitis, or by surgical trauma, appear to have two phases which have considerable clinical relevance. Animal studies[41] indicate that there is an acute peritonitis associated with a septicaemia, which has an appreciable mortality. The septicaemia usually appears to be due to aerobic organisms such as *E. coli*. Those animals which survive will then go on to form abscesses and it seems that the anaerobes are the organisms responsible for this phase of the disease. This does not mean that it is *only* the aerobes that are responsible for the early stages of infection and only the anaerobes for later abscess formation. Both groups of bacteria seem to be necessary and it is suggested that bacterial synergism plays a major role in this infection.

Multiple aerobes and anaerobes can be isolated from cases of peritonitis or from the abscesses. Therefore, how does one judge the relative importance of either group? The lowest mortality rates are seen if therapy is directed against the aerobe in the early stage of infection. If then anti-anaerobe therapy is begun there will be a low incidence of abscess formation. The best results are obtained by the use of combined therapy (Table 4). Such combinations might be gentamicin (or tobramycin) plus metronidazole or clindamycin. These regimes are now the mainstay of the therapy of intra-abdominal sepsis. The new cephamycin, cefoxitin, which is active against many anaerobes as well as common aerobes is proving to be effective monotherapy[29].

Table 4 Incidence of mortality and intra-abdominal abscess formation in experimental intra-abdominal infection in rats

Treatment group	Mortality		Abscess*	
	No.†	%	No.‡	%
Untreated control	22/60	37	38/38	100
Gentamicin	2/57	4	54/55	98
Clindamycin	21/60	35	2/39	5
Gentamicin + clindamycin	5/58	7	3/53	6

* Incidence of abscess formation when sacrificed at 2 weeks
† Number of fatalities/number studied
‡ Number with abscess/number studied
(from Finegold *et al.*[12])

The subphrenic area is the most common site for abscesses and the appendix is the commonest site of origin in this infection. Infections of the biliary tract, diverticulitis and leaking suture lines after bowel anastomosis are also common sites from which subphrenic abscesses arise. The subhepatic and paracolic areas are also common sites for abscess formation. Retroperitoneal abscesses may owe their origin to the kidney, pancreatic infections or the pleural space (as a psoas abscess).

Abscess formation in the liver is closely linked to anaerobic bacteria, and from over one half of abscesses in this organ anaerobes (most commonly *B. fragilis*) can be isolated[42]. As with any abscess, drainage is required which can be either aspiration or open, the former possibly having fewer complications. Metronidazole together with an aminoglycoside seems to be appropriate.

Anaerobic infections of the biliary tree are rare and the acute gaseous cholecystitis is most often seen in elderly diabetics. Clostridia are the commonest isolates from these patients. Anaerobes have been cultured from only 1–2% of diseased gall bladders and are a rare cause of cholecystitis.

Wound infections after surgery on the abdominal viscera are, unfortunately, all too common. Yet again the bacteria isolated reflect the bowel flora and *B. fragilis* is the commonest anaerobe isolated. Abdominal wall infections can range from a rather red wound through a smelly purulent discharge to frank dehiscence of the suture line. Rarely more spectacular infections may occur. We have seen several examples of Meleney's synergistic gangrene following lower bowel surgery from which anaerobic streptococci and staphylococci have been cultured. Gas gangrene is, mercifully, rare. The treatment of wound infections is very variable. Minor infections often need little in the way of specific therapy while a severe infection may need combined antimicrobials and often a recourse to further surgery.

Female genital tract
Anaerobes have been implicated in a very wide range of infections of the female genital tract including infections of the endometrium, myometrium, pelvic infections (and consequent peritonitis), wound infections, vulvar and Bartholin's gland abscess, vaginitis, salpingitis and tubo-ovarian abscess, septic abortion and infections of the neonate. After the gonococcus, anaerobes are the most important pathogens and *Bacteroides* spp., in particular *B. fragilis,* the most commonly isolated anaerobes[43]. Peptococci and peptostreptococci are also important. *Clostridium* spp. are important pathogens in septic abortion cases.

Post-hysterectomy
The majority of hysterectomies are now performed by the vaginal approach. This means that the operation is in a 'dirty' field. It is, therefore, not surprising that post-operative infections are common. This may just be an infection of the vaginal cuff – although pelvic abscess and cellulitis can occur. Drainage and appropriate chemotherapy (such as metronidazole) will usually cause rapid resolution. There is a good case for prophylactic administration of antimicrobials in this field.

Tubo-ovarian abscess
These infections are often related to previous operations on the female genital tract. As always in female genital tract infections a high vaginal swab is not a reliable guide in diagnosing possible infections of the adnexa. A swab taken at operation or at culdoscopy is required. After

this anti-microbial therapy combined with surgery is indicated and gentamicin plus metronidazole or clindamycin would be appropriate.

Endometritis

Infections of the uterus which may go on to pyometra are not uncommon where there is a cervical blockage such as in carcinoma of the cervix. Obviously in such cases treatment has to be directed at promoting drainage and unless there is evidence of pelvic cellulitis antibiotics have but a small part to play.

Vulvovaginal infections

Anaerobic infections of the vulva and vagina are most commonly vulval abscess and infected Bartholin's cyst. Anaerobic streptococci make up the majority of infecting organisms. Treatment is primarily surgical drainage.

Septic abortion

A very wide variety of organisms have been cultured from specimens taken in this important condition[33]. In one third of cases multiple organisms have been isolated, anaerobes in two thirds of cases and aerobes only in half. *Bacteroides* spp. and *Fusobacterium* are the commonest anaerobes and *E. coli* the commonest aerobe. About one third of patients have a concomitant bacteraemia, again emphasising the need to take blood cultures routinely. The usual treatment is dilation and curettage together with appropriate antibacterial cover, such as gentamicin or a cephalosporin plus metronidazole or clindamycin.

Overshadowing these more common infections is the spectre of clostridial sepsis which is usually associated with criminal abortions. This rapidly fatal condition is fortunately rare. The diagnosis may be suspected from the history, evidence of toxaemia, collapse and disseminated intravascular coagulation. Jaundiced serum is a poor prognostic sign. Treatment cannot wait for bacteriological confirmation and radical surgery, probably hysterectomy, together with large dose penicillin therapy are necessary.

It should be remembered that the isolation of a *Clostridium* sp. from a normal vagina, or from a case of mild infection is not uncommon, and even the isolation from cases of septic abortion does not mean that the patient has clostridial sepsis. The diagnosis is essentially clinical.

Amnionitis and post-partum infections

Amnionitis is usually associated with prolonged ruptured membranes and is usually caused by infection of the liquor by vaginal commensals, *E. coli, Bacteroides,* streptococci. The same organisms can cause post-partum infections of the endometrium. This is usually only a mild illness with fever and some increase in lochia and often settles down quite quickly. Occasionally evidence of spreading infection may be seen with chills, rigors, leukocytosis and abdominal pain. A foul smelling discharge may point to anaerobes as the infecting organisms. Treatment in amnionitis should be to expedite delivery and in severe post-partum sepsis, chemotherapy should be directed at the appropriate agent, found following a well taken specimen (an endo-cervical swab at least).

Bacteraemia

Over the last few years, the importance of anaerobes isolated from blood cultures has been realised. The incidence of anaerobic bacteraemia is extremely variable, but has been reported as high as 25% of all isolates[44]. There are many reasons for this variation such as laboratory methods, the groups of patients studied, the use of antibiotics at time of surgery etc., but most of all the awareness of the clinician of anaerobic sepsis and the frequency with which blood cultures are routinely taken. The anaerobe usually originates from an infection in the pelvis or abdomen. The 'Gram-negative' shock syndrome may well accompany the septicaemia and later metastatic abscess formation may occur.

It is important to realise that about one quarter to one third of patients with anaerobic bacteraemia will die – and this proportion will rise if more than one organism is isolated from the blood culture. By far the commonest anaerobe is *B. fragilis* and in some centres this is the second commonest pathogen from all blood cultures, *E. coli* being the organism most frequently isolated. In a recent review of the subject[45] it seems that the outcome was related more to the physical condition of the patient rather than whether antibiotic therapy was appropriate or not. Shock or oliguria were poor indicators of prognosis. Patients who were well enough to withstand surgery in order to drain an abscess, which was probably the portal of entry of the anaerobe into the blood, did well. Those patients who could not withstand such surgery did badly.

The poor prognosis should not of course mean that vigorous antimicrobial therapy should not be instituted. Metronidazole in combination with an aminoglycoside or cefoxitin alone are probably the best agents when anaerobic bacteraemia is suspected or the causative organism unknown. Therapy can be altered when the laboratory results have been reported.

It should be remembered that anaerobes can be isolated from blood culture bottles but the patient does not have an anaerobic bacteraemia; in other words contaminants have been reported. The commonest are *Propionibacterium* (a common skin commensal) and *Cl. perfringens,* an occasional visitor to skin especially if there is any faecal soiling (such as may occur if the blood culture has been taken by femoral artery puncture). This does not mean that these organisms are always only contaminants.

Soft tissue infections

A large variety of anaerobic soft tissue infections can occur. These are usually the result of some other problem such as trauma, vascular insufficiency, diabetes mellitus or foreign body. They rarely occur *de novo* and the therapy is usually difficult, requiring as a rule chemotherapy and surgery.

Gas gangrene is the most dramatic of the anaerobic bacterial diseases, but other anaerobes can cause soft tissue sepsis which at times can be just as difficult to treat.

(a) *Gas gangrene* – This disease is more correctly known as clostridial myonecrosis and is caused by one of the histotoxic clostridia becoming implanted in a wound (usually after trauma). *Cl. perfringens* is the commonest, but others encountered are *Cl. septicum, Cl. histolyticum,* and *Cl. novyi (oedematiens).* If the conditions in the tissues are suitable for the organism to multiply, a histotoxin may be elaborated. A low oxygen tension, as found in patients with vascular disease or in injuries causing devitalisation of tissue are important prerequisites. The usual preceding event for gas gangrene occurring in hospital is amputation of a lower limb, when the clostridium is assumed[46] to have come from the bowel of the patient. The organism may also come from the environment in traumatic injury where it may be existing as a spore changing into the vegetative form in the wound. The toxins produced can destroy tissue.

Lecithinases (the *a* toxins of *Cl. perfringens*) can destroy cell membranes. A toxin from *Cl. histolyticum* can digest tissues readily. The toxins will diffuse out from the point of infection, kill more tissue and so enable the dividing bacteria to move in. The toxins will also be absorbed into the blood stream and account for some of the clinical features of the disease. The production of gas occurs relatively late in the disease and may track up the tissue planes.

The clinical features can be very variable. The incubation period is usually a matter of hours to a day or two – but can be up to six weeks. The onset is often acute with severe pain and swelling of the affected area. The symptoms of the toxaemia are often pronounced. Patients are pale, ill, sweating, may be delirious and often have a tachycardia. Lecithinase activity can cause haemolysis and jaundice and these would be very grave prognostic signs as would shock or evidence of blood stream invasion. Evidence of gas, such as crepitus, is not very frequent although there may be radiological evidence if this is sought.

From what has been said about this notable condition it can be seen that the diagnosis must be a clinical one and prevention in this case is far more important than treatment ·(see this Chapter under heading Prophylaxis). The mainstay of therapy is adequate surgery. All affected tissue must be removed, tissue oxygenation being improved if necessary by laying open the area. By increasing the oxygen partial pressure the production of toxin will cease, but the toxin will not be neutralised. The use of hyperbaric oxygen in achieving this is of considerable interest although the results are open to question[47] [48]. The usual procedure is to expose the patient to three atmospheres pressure for periods up to 2 hours and repeating this five times in 48 hours. There are no controlled studies to confirm the efficacy of this treatment, which is understandable in a severe illness such as ̇his. The weight of opinion does favour the use of hyperbaric oxygen, even though it is not without risk to patient and attendants, i.e. aseptic bone necrosis and decompression sickness.

Antibiotics have a relatively little role to play in what is essentially a toxaemia. They should though be employed and penicillin, 10–20 mega units per day, is recommended. The value of antitoxin remains unproved although in the early stages of the disease there may be some benefit[49].

(b) *Synergistic bacterial gangrene* – This is the rare disease described by Meleney[50], that typically begins at the site of a surgical drain or near sutures and spreads as a black necrotic area around which there is an area of oedematous erythema. Although routine culture from the slough may yield only coliforms, from the advancing edge two synergistic pathogens should be isolated, a microaerophilic streptococcus and *Staph. aureus*. The treatment is extensive debridement plus local treatment with gauze soaked in neomycin and bacitracin. High dose antistaphylococcal therapy with flucloxacillin or clindamycin should also be started.

Necrotising fasciitis
This is a rare but serious infection the pathogenesis of which has only recently been discovered. It is an infection of the superficial fascia which causes widespread necrosis and undermining of the surrounding tissues. It often follows trauma or surgery and the initial injury may be quite trivial – insect bites or bruises. From the serosanguinous pus a variety of pathogens may be isolated, such as β-*haemolytic streptococci, Staph. aureus* and coliforms. In most cases careful bacteriology will yield either a *Peptostreptococcus, Bacteroides* or a *Fusobacterium*. The

last two are usually found together with a coliform[51]. Therapy should be prompt and radical excision with drainage together with massive doses of appropriate antimicrobials.

Prophylaxis of anaerobic infections

Enthusiasm as to the role of prophylaxis against all infections appears to wax and wane with time and place. On the one hand all would agree that prevention is better than cure but on the other antibiotics can be a menace to the patient and his environment. The increased use of antibiotics is almost certainly associated with the appearance of bacterial antimicrobial resistance. Many would argue that successful agents such as cefoxitin and metronidazole should not be used in the prophylaxis of anaerobic infections lest their useful life be shortened. At present there is no evidence that this will occur but there is ample evidence of aerobes becoming resistant, causing considerable clinical problems which do not disappear until the antibiotic in question is withdrawn. Such considerations as to long term problems are not readily appreciated by many clinicians. What is of more immediate concern to them is if the antibiotic is positively dangerous to the patient. A very good example of this is the problem of pseudomembranous colitis which may follow any antimicrobial administration but is most often seen after using clindamycin or lincomycin. In one study[52] a number of patients, some of whom had only received antibiotics for 24 hours for prophylaxis in bowel surgery, developed this condition and one third of those died. A clinician's approach to prophylaxis using antibiotics should therefore be guarded and, as is often the case, one tends to compromise. The rule is: if antibiotics are to be given for the prophylaxis of infection they should be used for the shortest period of time.

In some circumstances antibiotic prophylaxis is mandatory. Amputations of the lower limb and hip operations, as has already been mentioned, carry a definite risk of contamination with *Cl. perfringens* from the bowel flora of the patient, and then possible gas gangrene. This risk is increased in diabetics. It is common practice to use prophylactic penicillin starting just before the operation and continuing for five days. A useful adjuvant to this is the adequate preparation of the operation site with povidone-iodine compresses which greatly reduce the numbers of *Cl. perfringens* present[46].

The main area of contention over the prophylactic use of antibiotics in association with anaerobic infections is in bowel surgery. Operations on the large bowel carry a high rate of infection and morbidity. Anything which will reduce this is obviously desirable and efficient. Surgeons should remember that the large bowel cannot be 'sterilised'. Mechanical or antibiotic preparation can at best only reduce the bacterial load which will spill from an opened viscus. Careful surgical technique is far more important than 'sticking the patient on antibiotics'. Having said this, there is evidence that an agent active against anaerobes, such as metronidazole, will if given over the time of operation, cut down anaerobic sepsis[53]. There is also some information, most of it anecdotal, that in bowel and gynaecological surgery, if one administers an anti-microbial active against either an aerobe or anaerobe the incidence of infection due to either is reduced. Obviously a considerable amount of work is still yet to be done. What advice can be given until an answer is available? Clean surgery should not need any antibiotic prophylaxis. When operating upon contaminated sites (bowel or vagina) if prophylaxis is to be given this should be with a narrow spectrum anti-anaerobic agent (such as metronidazole) which is known to be non-toxic and, most importantly, the drug should only be given to cover the period of operation, i.e. one or two doses only.

References

1   Pasteur, L. (1861). *Comptes Rendus de l'Academe des Sciences,* **52,** 344
2   Pasteur, L. (1878). *Comptes Rendus de l'Academe des Sciences,* **86,** 1037
3   Kitasato, S. (1889). *Z. Hyg. Infektionskrankh.,* **7,** 225
4   Florey, M. E. and Cairns, H. (1943). *Investigation of War Wounds, Penicillins. Preliminary Report to War Office and Medical Research Council.* (W.O. Publication, AMD 7/90D/43)
5   Alston, J. M. (1955). Necrobacillosis in Great Britain. *Brit. Med. J.,* **2,** 1524
6   MacLennan, J. D. (1951). In J. H. Dible and J. D. MacLennan (eds.) *Recent Advances in Bacteriology,* Chapter 2. (London: Churchill)
7   Gillespie, W. A. and Guy, J. (1956). Bacteroides in intra-abdominal sepsis: their sensitivity to antibiotics. *Lancet,* **1,** 1039
8   Gunn, A. A. (1956). Bacteroides septicaemia. *J. R. Coll. Surgeons (Edin.),* **2,** 41
9   Hilstead, A. G., Kimbull, J. M. and Maki, D. G. (1977). Recovery of anaerobic, facultative and aerobic bacteria from clinical specimens. *J. Clin. Microbiol.,* **5,** 564
10 Gorbach, S. L. (1971). Intestinal microflora. *Gastroenterology,* **60,** 1110
11 Hill, M. J. and Drasar, B. S. (1974). In A. Barlows (ed.) *Anaerobic Bacteria Role in Disease,* p. 119. (Springfield, Ill: Charles C. Thomas)
12 Finegold, S. M., Bartlett, J. G., Chow, A. W., Flora, D. J., Gorbach, S. L., Harder, E. J. and Tally, F. P. (1975). Management of anaerobic infections. *Ann. Int. Med.,* **83,** 375
13 Fildes, P. (1929). Tetanus: The oxidation reduction potential of subcutaneous tissue fluid. *Brit. J. Exp. Pathol.,* **10,** 197
14 Mergerhagen, S. E., Thonard, J. C. and Scherp, H. W. (1958). Studies on synergistic infection. *J. Infect. Dis.,* **103,** 33
15 MacDonald, J. B., Socransky, S. S. and Gibbon, S. R. J. (1963). Aspects of the pathogenesis of mixed anaerobic infections of mucous membranes. *J. Dent. Res.,* **42,** 529
16 Ingham, H. R., Sisson, P. R., Tharagonnet, D., Selkon, J. B. and Codd, A. A. (1977). Inhibition of phagocytosis *in vitro* by obligate anaerobes. *Lancet,* **2,** 1252
17 Weinrich, A. E. and DelBene, V. E. (1976). β-lactamase activity in anaerobic bacteria. *Antimicrob. Agents Chemother.,* **10,** 106

18 O'Keefe, J. P., Tally, F. P., Barza, M. and Gorbach, S. L. (1978). Inactivation of penicillin G during experimental infections with *B. fragilis*. *J. Infect. Dis.*, **137**, 437

19 Fiedelman, W. and Webb, C. C. (1975). Clinical evaluation of carbenicillin in the treatment of infections due to anaerobic species. *Curr. Ther. Res.*, **18**, 441

20 Hunter, P. A. and Reading, C. (1976). Sodium clavulanate, a novel and potent β-lactamase inhibitor. Presented at the *16th Inter-science Conference on Antimicrobial Agents and Chemotherapy*, October 27–29, Chicago

21 Wise, R. (1976). Clavulanic acid and susceptibility of *B. fragilis* to penicillin. *Lancet*, **2**, 145

22 Bartlett, J. G., Onderdonk, A. B., Cisneros, R. L. and Kasper, D. L. (1977). Clindamycin associated colitis due to a toxin producing species of *Clostridia* in hamsters. *J. Infect. Dis.*, **136**, 701

23 Tally, F. P., Snydman, D. R., Gorbach, S. L. and Malamy, M. H. (1978). Plasmid-mediated transferable clindamycin resistance in *Bacteroides fragilis*. Presented at the *18th Interscience Conference on Antimicrobial Agents and Chemotherapy*, October 1–4, Atlanta

24 Ingham, H. R., Eaton, S., Venables, C. W. and Adams, P. C. (1978). *B. fragilis* resistance to metronidazole after long term therapy. *Lancet*, **1**, 214

25 Willis, A. T., Jones, P. H., Phillips, K. D. and Gottobed, G. (1978). Metronidazole resistance among *B. fragilis*. *Lancet*, **1**, 721

26 Finegold, S. M. (1977). *Anaerobic bacteria in human diseases*, p. 545. (New York: Academic Press)

27 Louie, T. J., Bartlett, J. G., Onderdonk, A. B. and Gorbach, S. L. (1977). Failure of chloramphenicol therapy in experimental intra-abdominal abscess. Presented at the *17th Interscience Conference on Antimicrobial Agents and Chemotherapy*, October 12–14, New York

28 Ingham, H. R., Selkon, J. B., Codd, A. A. and Hale, J. H. (1970). The effect of carbon dioxide on the sensitivity of *B. fragilis* to certain antibiotics in vitro. *J. Clin. Pathol.*, **23**, 254

29 Geddes, A. M., Schnurr, L. P., Ball, A. P., McGhie, D., Brookes, G. R., Wise, R. and Andrews, J. M. (1977). Cefoxitin: a hospital study. *Brit. Med. J.*, **1**, 1126

30 Kerry, D. W., Hamilton-Miller, J. M. T. and Brumfitt, W. (1975). Trimethoprim and rifampicin: *in vitro* activities separately and in combination. *J. Antimicrob. Chemother.*, **1**, 417

31 Phillips, I. and Warren, C. (1975). Susceptibility of *B. fragilis* to spectinomycin. *J. Antimicrob. Chemother.*, **1**, 91

32 Finegold, S. M. (1977). *Anaerobic bacteria in human disease*, p. 231. (New York: Academic Press)

33 Finegold, S. M., Bartlett, J. G., Chow, A. W., Flora, D. J., Gorbach, S. L., Harder, E. J. and Tally, F. P. (1975). Management of anaerobic infections. *Ann. Int. Med.*, **83**, 375

34 Heineman, H. S. and Braude, A. I. (1963). Anaerobic infections of the brain. *Am. J. Med.*, **35**, 682

35 de Louvois, J. and Hurley, R. (1975). Antibiotic concentrations in intracranial pus. *Chemotherapy*, **4**, 61

36 Barting, R. W. A. and Selkon, J. B. (1978). Penetration of antibiotics into CSF and brain tissue. *J. Antimicrob. Chemother.*, **4**, 203

37 de Louvois, J., Gortvai, P. and Hurley, R. (1977). Antibiotic treatment of abscesses of the CNS. *Brit. Med. J.*, **2**, 985

38 Headington, J. T. and Beyerlein, B. (1966). Anaerobic bacteria in routine urine culture. *J. Clin. Pathol.*, **19**, 573

39 Swenson, R. M., Lorber, B., Michaelson, T. C. and Spalding, E. H. (1974). The bacteriology of intra-abdominal infections. *Arch. Surg.*, **109**, 398

40 Gorbach, S. L., Thadepalli, H. and Norsen, J. (1972). Microorganisms in intra-abdominal infections. Presented at the *International Conference on Anaerobic Bacteria*, November 27–29, Atlanta

41 Weinstein, W. M., Onderdonk, A. B., Bartlett, J. G., Louie, T. J. and Gorbach, S. L. (1975). Antimicrobial therapy of experimental intra-abdominal sepsis. *J. Infect. Dis.*, **132**, 282

42 Sabbaj, J., Sutter, V. L. and Finegold, S. M. (1972). Anaerobic pyogenic liver abscess. *Ann. Int. Med.*, **77**, 629

43 Gorbach, S. L. and Bartlett, J. C. (1974). Anaerobic infections. *New Engl. J. Med.*, **290**, 1177

44 Wilson, W. R., Martin, M. J., Wilkowske, C. J. and Washington, J. A. (1972). Anaerobic bacteraemia. *Mayo Clinic Proceedings*, **47**, 639

45 Washington, J. A. (1978). Treatment of bacteraemia due to anaerobic bacteria. *J. Antimicrob. Chemother.* (In press.)

46 Ayliffe, G. A. J. and Lowbury, E. J. L. (1966). Sources of gas gangrene in hospital. *Brit. Med. J.*, **2**, 333

47 Weinstein, L. and Barza, M. A. (1973). Gas gangrene. *New. Engl. J. Med.*, **289**, 1129

48 Leading Article. (1972). Gas gangrene and hyperbaric oxygen. *Brit. Med. J.*, **3**, 715

49 MacLennan, J. D., (1962). The histotoxic clostridial infections of man. *Bacteriol. Rev.*, **26**, 177

50 Meleney, F. L. (1931). Progressive gangrenous infection. *Ann. Surg.*, **94**, 961

51 Menda, K. B., Norsen, J., Kallick, C., *et al.* (1974). Necrotising fasciitis. Abstract *14th Inter-science Conference on Antimicrobial Agents and Chemotherapy*, San Francisco

52 Clarke, C. E., Thompson, H., McLeish, A. R., Powis, S. J. A., Dorricott, N. J. and Alexander-Williams, J. (1976). Pseudomembranous colitis following prophylactic antibiotics in bowel surgery. *J. Antimicrob. Chemother.*, **2**, 167

53 Study Group. (1975). An evaluation of metronidazole in the prophylaxis and treatment of anaerobic infections in surgical patients. *J. Antimicrob. Chemother.*, **1**, 393

54 McCord, J. M., Keele, B. B. and Fridovich, I. (1971). An enzyme based theory of obligate anaerobiosis. *Proc. Natl. Acad. Sci. USA*, **68**, 1024

5

The chemotherapy of gonorrhoea and non-specific genital infections

G. L. Ridgway

INTRODUCTION

The spectrum of sexually transmitted diseases has changed in recent years[1]. No longer is the physician dealing with two diseases (gonorrhoea and syphilis) treatable with a single antibiotic (penicillin). Chlamydiae, mycoplasmas, other bacteria (Donovan's bacillus, *Haemophilus ducreyii,* anaerobes), viruses, protozoa, fungi and arthropods may all be encountered, often not alone in any individual patient. Willcox[2][3] has ably reviewed the attitude of the pharmaceutical industry to this range of organisms, drawing attention to a number of deficiencies, both in the provision of established antibiotics (e.g. depot penicillin preparations), and failure to achieve satisfactory chemotherapy for some diseases (*Herpes genitalis*).

Until recently the chemotherapy of sexually transmitted diseases has been restricted to a few well tried antibiotics. Within the last few years, however, the results of both clinical and research work have led to a reappraisal of current treatment regimens. The gonococcus has shown decreasing sensitivity to penicillin for a number of years, but the emergence of the β-lactamase-producing strains, though predicted[4], caused consternation, as penicillin will not cure infections with these strains. The establishment of *Chlamydia trachomatis* as a cause of 50–60% of non-gonococcal urethritis in men[5][6] has allowed rationalisation of treatment for this very common disease. For syphilis treatment penicillin is universally used, but recent work has cast doubts on long-term cure with conventional doses of this antibiotic, owing to the demonstration of treponeme-like forms in the cerebro-spinal fluid (CSF) in patients previously treated with penicillin[7], and low levels of penicillin in the CSF[8] after therapy particularly with benzathine penicillin. Rapid advances by the pharmaceutical industry have resulted in the marketing of a bewildering number of new antibiotics applicable to gonorrhoea and non-specific genital infections (NSGI). Sometimes these are merely expensive modifications of existing, established antimicrobials, but some now have a place in the therapy of the sexually transmitted diseases.

The clinician dealing with these infections is confronted with two broad groups of diseases. Firstly, those that have a readily identifiable cause, e.g. gonorrhoea, where the success of therapy can be judged by the eradication of the infecting organism, or secondly, the so-called 'non-specific' infections, where a definite cause is either not known, or not readily identifiable. In this latter group, treatment may of necessity be with less satisfactory empirical regimens; in this field major advances in aetiology have recently been made.

In order to give patients the benefit of specific treatment when indicated, the clinician must provide the microbiologist with good quality, relevant specimens. Any result from the laboratory can only reflect the material on which the tests were performed. Specimens from all potentially infected sites should be collected for examination by microscopy and/or culture, and for some diseases, e.g. syphilis, serological tests are mandatory. The exact technique for processing specimens will vary between laboratories, and the clinician should be aware of the local methods for transporting and storing specimens.

CHEMOTHERAPY OF GONORRHOEA

The chemotherapy of gonorrhoea requires a drug fulfilling a number of criteria. An effective drug must work in a single dose, and be rapidly bactericidal. Adequate blood levels maintained for 8–12 h should eliminate the gonococcus, which thus lends itself to such single dose therapy. The use of multidose regimens in uncomplicated gonorrhoea involves patient compliance in the cure; this compliance is often hard to achieve in the field of sexually transmitted diseases. For similar reasons, many physicians prefer injectable to oral preparations. The antibiotic should be cheap, as large scale usage will be necessary, particularly in developing countries. Side effects, be they toxic, allergenic, or microbiogenic, should not occur. The emergence of resistance should not be a feature of the antimicrobial agent. Patients with one sexually transmitted disease such as gonorrhoea may also be incubating another, syphilis being the most important. It has therefore been advocated that an ideal anti-gonococcal agent should be inactive against *Treponema pallidum*, so that the diagnosis of syphilis is not obscured. Some authorities, however, suggest that regimens for treating gonorrhoea should also abort incubating syphilis, to the advantage of the patient[2]. Upwards of 40% of men with acute gonococcal urethritis will present with a persistent urethritis after adequate pencillin therapy – post-gonococcal urethritis (PGU). This is almost certainly due to the acquisition of both the gonococcus and an agent of NGU at the same time. In women, a situation analogous to PGU in men may persist after treatment for gonorrhoea, leading to an unrecognised reservoir for transmission of NGU to subsequent male partners. Consequently, treatment for gonorrhoea should ideally eradicate organisms causing NGU. Owing to the risk of inducing resistance in other organisms, the antibiotic chosen should not be in use for the therapy of life threatening diseases. There is a wide variation in resistance patterns of *Neisseria gonorrhoeae* throughout the world, so therapy must be modified in the light of local sensitivity patterns. A failure rate of greater than 5% for gonococcal urethritis should lead to a reappraisal of treatment schedules.

Until the advent of the sulphonamides in 1937[9] previous remedies had been with non-specific agents. But early success with these drugs was soon marred by the emergence of resistance, to the extent that when penicillin was introduced in the 1940's, 75% of gonococcal strains were resistant to sulphonamides. With the establishment of penicillin for therapy, has come increasing resistance to not only penicillin but ampicillin, streptomycin, erythromycin, tetracycline, and cephaloridine.

Needless to say, the ideal drug does not exist, and even penicillin which comes closest to the ideal is under a cloud, due to the development of resistance, both partial over the last 30 years, and total with the emergence of β-lactamase-producing gonococci.

Penicillins
The penicillins remain the mainstay of treatment. Originally, 150 000 units of a repository penicillin was adequate for cure. Now, at least 2.4 megaunits of aqueous procaine penicillin G plus probenecid is required in Europe. In North America, the Center for Disease Control recommends 4.8 megaunits of procaine penicillin plus probenecid, and similar dosage is in use in Africa, India and the Far East. Slow release preparations of penicillin (e.g. Benzathine or PAM), or the oral penicillins such as penicillin V (phenoxymethyl penicillin) are best avoided for single dose therapy owing to variations in absorption. An alternative parenteral single dose therapy is to use 5 megaunits (3 g) of

benzyl penicillin, dissolved in 8 ml of 0.5% lignocaine given intramuscularly, along with 1 g of probenecid orally[10]. Ideally, probenecid should be given 30 minutes before a parenteral dose of penicillin. These parenteral regimens approach the maximum tolerable amount of penicillin that can be injected intramuscularly. The use of procaine or lignocaine introduces another potentially toxic agent into the therapy, along with probenecid, which may precipitate acute gout in susceptible patients, and the allergenic properties of penicillin itself. Even these massive doses will be ineffective against the recently described β-lactamase producing strains of *N. gonorrhoeae*.

For the oral treatment of gonorrhoea, the semisynthetic penicillins have proved useful. Ampicillin is now well established in therapy, although as with penicillins, regimens vary with resistance patterns. Probenecid is used concurrently, and has prolonged the useful life of both penicillin and other semisynthetic penicillins in gonorrhoea. A number of studies with ampicillin have been reported. Groth and Hallquist[11] found a 2 g dose of ampicillin, plus 1 g of probenecid, both administered orally, to be effective; Bro-Jorgensen and Jensen[12] found this regimen to be better than ampicillin alone, noting that the probenecid could be given at the same time as the ampicillin. Two excellent studies by Eriksson[13 14] confirmed this regimen for uncomplicated gonorrhoea in men and women, again noting the inferiority of 2 g ampicillin alone. In the Phillipines, Kvale *et al.*[15] found that 3.5 g of ampicillin plus probenecid was necessary, and this regimen has been adopted by the CDC, preferably for use only in patients who refuse parenteral penicillin therapy. In England, the 2 g ampicillin plus 1 g probenecid regimen still appears to give satisfactory results in uncomplicated gonorrhoea in men and women.

Newer esters of ampicillin have now been produced, and these have had a varied reception. Willcox[16] found that amoxycillin in a dose of less than 2 g gave an unacceptably high failure rate; in a dose of 2 g plus 1 g probenecid, with a further dose of probenecid at 5 hours, the failure rate was still 10%. Better results have been obtained with 3 g of amoxycillin, with and without probenecid[17 19]. These treatments seem to have little advantage over conventional therapy with ampicillin/probenecid.

Talampicillin, which is hydrolysed to ampicillin after absorption, is a newer addition to the semisynthetic penicillins. Willcox[20] reported encouraging results using 1.5 g of talampicillin without probenecid, demonstrating a 95.8% rate of cure.

The National gonorrhoea monitoring study[21] reported in 1976, compared four standard regimens (as recommended by the United States Public Health Service in 1972). Over 9000 patients were treated in this study, randomly assigned to one of the following: 4.8 megaunits of aqueous procaine penicillin plus 1 g probenecid, 3.5 g ampicillin plus 1 g of probenecid, 1.5 g tetracycline hydrochloride followed by 2 g daily for four days, or 2 g intramuscularly of spectinomycin dihydrochloride (4 g in women). The cure rates were 96.8% for procaine penicillin, and 92.8, 96.2, and 92.8% for the other regimens respectively. All four regimens were noted to be effective, but the significant difference between the procaine penicillin and ampicillin regimens was stressed.

Some physicians advocate the use of larger doses when treating women, but there is no evidence to support this.

For the last thirty years, the increasing resistance to penicillin by the gonococcus has been stepwise through chromosomal mutation and genetic selection, remaining within the bounds of clinically attainable blood levels. In 1976, Phillips[22] described a strain of *N. gonorrhoeae* isolated in London, which produced a β-lactamase enzyme. Simultaneously, Ashford *et al.*[23] reported a similar strain from California. Organisms of this type are totally resistant to all the penicillins, and to the majority of the cephalosporins. Early fears of the widespread appearance of these strains have not been realised, except in a few areas, such as the Phillipines and S.E. Asia. There is at present no need to abandon penicillin or ampicillin as the first line treatment. However, it is essential that all patients suspected of suffering from gonorrhoea have relevant cultures performed, and that all isolates are screened for penicillin resistance. Evidence suggests that the plasmid is easily lost[24], and consequently these strains are unlikely to become dominant.

A single dose regimen is not recommended for gonorrhoea in sites other than the cervix or urethra. A number of regimens may be considered, however, if outpatient treatment is contemplated, then close follow-up must be applied. A suitable in-patient regimen is an injection of 5 megaunits of benzyl penicillin plus 1 g of probenecid orally as a starter dose, followed by an injection of 1 megaunit benzyl penicillin 6-hourly with 1 g of probenecid 12-hourly for a total of 10 days. For outpatient or oral treatment, an initial dose of 3.5 g of ampicillin plus 1 g of probenecid is followed by 1 g of ampicillin 6-hourly with probenecid 1 g 12-hourly for a total of 10 days.

Pharyngeal gonorrhoea appears particularly resistant to penicillin therapy. Procaine penicillin (4.8 megaunits) plus probenecid may be effective, but an alternative antimicrobial, such as doxycycline should be used.

Gonococcal ophthalmia neonatorum is still best treated with penicillin. Local penicillin (250 i.u.) should be instilled every minute for the first 15 minutes, with saline irrigations, increasing to hourly for the first 24 hours. Systemic penicillin should also be prescribed (100 000 i.u. 12-hourly for 5 days).

Cephalosporins

The cephalosporins have proved disappointing. They are painful to inject. Because of cross allergenicity to the penicillins, they should not be used as substitutes. Keys et al.[25] obtained an 84% cure with 2 g of cephaloridine for urethral gonorrhoea in men. Willcox[26] used 2 g of cephalexin (an oral preparation), followed by a further 2 g of cephalexin 6 h later. A 14.6% failure rate was recorded.

Cefuroxime, a new β-lactamase-stable cephalosporin, shows possible potential against β-lactamase-producing gonococci. Arya et al.[27] working in Liverpool, used cefuroxime in a single dose of 1 g by intramuscular injection to treat seven women with β-lactamase-producing strains of N. gonorrhoeae, with no failures. A recent study by Fowler et al.[28] compared 3 dose regimens for gonorrhoea in men and women. A dose of 750 mg cefuroxime plus 1 g of probenecid gave cure rates over 90% for both sexes. A preliminary report by Xeri and Orsoloni[29] indicates that cefuroxime is treponemocidal. Further experience with this antibiotic is required.

Aminoglycosides

Streptomycin has fallen into disuse in the treatment of gonorrhoea. Initial success was overshadowed by the emergence of resistance. Resistance to streptomycin is linked to relative resistance to penicillin. Relative ototoxicity compared with other available antibiotics for gonorrhoea would further preclude the use of streptomycin today.

Kanamycin, though becoming increasingly difficult to obtain, has a place primarily because of its inactivity against T. pallidum. Garrod and Waterworth[30] noted the potentiation of penicillin and sulphafurazole by kanamycin against the gonococcus. A single dose injection of 2 g is effective.

Gentamicin, likewise, has no effect on incubating syphilis, however this is an important antibiotic for use in life-threatening diseases, and its widespread use for treating gonorrhoea is to be discouraged.

The aminoglycosides all have in common potential toxicity to both the eighth nerve, and the kidneys. In consequence, they should be used with caution in patients on diuretics, or with renal disease. They are cross-allergenic.

Spectinomycin

This antibiotic, an aminocyclitol, is closely related to the aminoglycosides. As it is effective in a single dose, and used almost solely in the treatment of gonorrhoea, this drug may well prove useful as the first line treatment of β-lactamase-producing gonococci. It has some activity against T. pallidum, and is not, therefore, a substitute for kanamycin.

Karney *et al.*[31] treated 971 men with anogenital gonorrhoea with 2 g of spectinomycin, with a failure rate of 6.3%. Using 4 g of spectinomycin on 951 men and 1016 women, the failure rate was 3.9% in each group. Pharyngeal gonorrhoea responded poorly. Porter and Rutherford[32] encountered one treatment failure among 75 patients with uncomplicated gonorrhoea treated with 2 g of spectinomycin. Resistant mutants can be selected *in vitro*, and have been encountered clinically[33] [34], hence the risk of emergence of resistant organisms with the widespread use of spectinomycin is very real. Its use should at present be restricted to patients intolerant of penicillin, or known to be harbouring β-lactamase-producing gonococci.

The macrolides
The macrolides have had a disappointing record in the treatment of gonorrhoea. Spiromycin seems to have fallen into disuse with unacceptable failure rates for both single- and multi-dose regimens. Erythromycin in a single dose has not proved to be effective, even with the more reliably absorbed stearate preparation. Brown *et al.*[35] recently compared the base and estolate in the treatment of gonococcal urethritis. A 9 g course was used, with 24% and 23% failure rates for base and estolate respectively. However, the safety of erythromycin in pregnancy is such that this antibiotic should be considered in pregnant women intolerant of penicillin. The recommended dose regimen of the CDC is 1.5 g orally, followed by 0.5 g 6-hourly for 4 days. The estolate should be avoided.

A newer addition to the macrolide range is rosamicin. *In vitro* studies[36] on 50 isolates of *N. gonorrhoeae* showed that 94% had a minimum inhibitory concentration of $0.03 \mu g/ml$. At this level, 46% of the isolates were sensitive to penicillin, 12% to erythromycin, and 6% to tetracycline. Results of clinical studies are awaited with interest.

Tetracycline
The tetracyclines have been widely used in the treatment of gonorrhoea. A large number of preparations are available, but in general there is little to choose between them. Oxytetracycline is the cheapest, and the most effective for general use. Absorption from the gastro-intestinal tract is good, but ideally tablets should be taken on an empty stomach. Calcium, iron, magnesium and bismuth will chelate with tetracyclines, preventing absorption. Milk, milk products, antacids and iron tablets should therefore be avoided during treatment. The calcium chelate is deposited in developing bones and teeth, consequently tetracyclines should not be prescribed to children under 12 years of age, or during pregnancy. Since the tetracyclines have a broad spectrum of activity, the normal flora may

be adversely affected, resulting in intestinal upset or candida overgrowth.

The results of therapy with single oral doses have proved variable, and the use of tetracyclines in this form cannot be recommended.

Karney *et al.*[31] reporting on a comparative study of tetracycline versus spectinomycin in 4043 patients with acute gonorrhoea, found a 94% cure rate with an initial 1.5 g dose of tetracycline followed by 500 mg 6-hourly for 4 days. This regimen is now recommended by CDC for penicillin-allergic patients. The loading dose is probably unnecessary. Resistance to the tetracyclines when found is partial, and cross resistance to streptomycin occurs. In the above study, failure of treatment was correlated with *in.vitro* resistance to tetracycline.

Newer tetracyclines, such as minocycline and doxycycline have been investigated. Masterton and Schofield[37] used a single dose of 300 mg or 400 mg of minocycline to treat 349 men with uncomplicated gonococcal urethritis. Failure rates of 3.2% and 5.1% respectively were obtained. Side effects were described as trivial. Parriser and Marino[38] treated 248 men with gonococcal urethritis, with a single 250 mg capsule of minocycline, and claimed a cure rate of between 69% and 92.5% depending on criteria for cure. Shahidullah[39] also using 300 mg of minocycline as a single dose recorded a cure rate of 94% in men.

Doxycycline has also produced variable results in single dose therapy, but has proved useful in the treatment of pharyngeal gonorrhoea using 200 mg as a starter dose, followed by 100 mg 12-hourly for 5 days.

The use of tetracyclines in the treatment of gonococcal urethritis consistently reduces the incidence of post-gonococcal urethritis, even with a single dose treatment. However, this must be balanced against a greater failure rate with gonorrhoea than other established single dose regimens.

Other antimicrobials

A great variety of antimicrobials have been investigated for anti-gonococcal activity. Those used as the mainstay of treatment are detailed above.

Chloramphenicol has been shown to be effective. Willcox[40] obtained a 95% cure using a single dose of 1 g. The potential toxicity of this agent, and its important uses in other diseases should prohibit its use in gonorrhoea. The less effective, and probably less toxic, synthetic alternative, thiamphenicol, is however in widespread use in continental Europe. A single dose of 2.5 g (10 × 250 mg capsules) is given orally. Failure rates of around 2.5% are claimed, and the dose probably does affect incubating syphilis[41].

Co-trimoxazole, a combination of sulphamethoxazole and

trimethoprim was shown by Csonka and Knight[42] to be effective in the therapy of gonorrhoea. Single dose studies have proved disappointing. Svinland[43] used four tablets twice daily for 2 days in both men and women with uncomplicated gonorrhoea, with failure rates of around 1%. Co-trimoxazole will not mask incubating syphilis, and in the dosage given would appear to have a place in the therapy of gonorrhoea when syphilis is suspected concurrently.

Rifampicin was used by Cobbold *et al.*[44] in a single oral dose of 900 mg to treat men with gonococcal urethritis. A failure rate of 11.2% was recorded. Results of others indicate that treatment failure may be due to emerging resistance.

Post-gonococcal urethritis responds to the antimicrobial agents used to treat NGU. There may well be a case for prospective treatment, using for example a standard penicillin treatment for the gonorrhoea, followed by a short course of a tetracycline.

The ideal antimicrobial for treating gonorrhoea has yet to be reported. The emergence of gonococci totally resistant to penicillin demonstrates that complacency with current schedules cannot be condoned. The geographical distribution of resistance patterns, coupled with epidemiological studies on gonococcal infections are necessary to allow the efficient use of antimicrobial agents currently available, and the evaluation of new agents.

THE CHEMOTHERAPY OF NON-SPECIFIC GENITAL INFECTIONS

In 1950, Harkness[45] described abacterial urethritis in men thus: "The prognosis is bad, but less gloomy than generally supposed." Cure was possible in 3–6 weeks with skilled local therapy. The treatment of choice was urethro-vesical irrigations with warm oxycyanate of mercury (1 : 4000 or 1 : 8000) augmented with weekly dilatation of the urethra. Writing only two years after the appearance of the tetracyclines, Harkness predicted that they could well become the treatment of choice.

Rational therapy of non-specific genital infection (NSGI) has been difficult in the past, owing to failure to confirm an aetiological agent for some or all cases. Therapy has been empirical, aided to a considerable extent by spontaneous resolution. The establishment of *Chlamydia trachomatis* as an aetiological agent in around 50% of cases of non-gonococcal urethritis (NGU)[5 6], has allowed some rationalisation of treatment regimens. However, since the role of other infecting organisms in NGU is undecided, in at least 50% of cases empirical treatment is unavoidable.

Holmes *et al.*[46] drew attention to the shortcomings of many empirical clinical trials in NGU with the following points:

(1) Reliance upon the examining physician's subjective evaluation in establishing the diagnosis of NGU, and in classifying patients as 'failures' or 'cures' following treatment

(2) Inadequate experimental controls, and failure to use a double blind design in treatment and follow-up examination

(3) Reliance upon patients self-administering medication without supervision

(4) Inability to prevent sexual re-exposure and possible re-infection of patients following treatment

(5) Incomplete follow-up, with compilation of treatment results based only on the progressively diminishing proportion of patients who return for follow-up.

Correction of many of these points is impractical outside the confines of the aircraft carrier used in their study. Unless there are rigidly applied and generally accepted criteria for what constitutes cure, the comparison of different treatments, or the same regimen in different parts of the world is impossible. A major epidemiological disadvantage of the purely clinical evaluation of therapy is that an observer cannot discern whether or at what point the patient had become non-infectious to others. This is of particular importance in the case of chlamydial NGU, since *C. trachomatis* is an important pathogen in women.

Placebo controlled trials have shown that approximately 60% of patients will have undergone spontaneous resolution after 3 months. If patients are evaluated during the first month after placebo therapy, however, the clinical response is unacceptably low. Holmes *et al.*[46] found that 14% of the men with NGU responded to placebo; in the discussion to that paper, four other trials are described, with cure rates ranging from zero to 28% after 7 days of placebo, rising to 71% in one trial after 28 days. An extensive evaluation of many antimicrobials by Willcox[47] showed placebo to be effective in about 30% (although duration of follow-up and criteria of cure are not recorded). This success rate was equivalent to that found with ampicillin, nalidixic acid, and novobiocin. Other compounds in this study of questionable value (greater than 37% failure rate) included sulphonamides alone, penicillin, chloramphenicol, streptomycin, metronidazole and spectinomycin. The above findings are reflected in the relative inactivity of these agents against *C. trachomatis in vitro*[48 49]. However, Holmes *et al.*[46] demonstrated beyond question that in the short term, tetracycline therapy was greatly superior to a placebo. In clinical practice today, effective antimicrobials have been narrowed down to the tetracyclines, erythromycin, and sulphonamide plus streptomycin. Rifampicin, highly effective against *C. trachomatis in vitro*, has curiously not been reported in controlled trials on NGU, although there is some evidence that resistance is readily inducible to this antibiotic[50]. Combination therapy (1 g of streptomycin as a single intramuscular injection, followed by 5 or 6 g of a soluble sulphonamide daily in divided doses for 5 days) must now be regarded as obsolete.

There are a large number of tetracyclines available. Almost all have been or are used in the therapy of NGU. To this must be added the permutations of dose and duration to produce the current confused state on ideal therapy. Comparative studies have taken little account of the pharmacokinetics of the tetracyclines. The problems of empirical studies were well highlighted by Simopoulos[51]. It is only comparatively recently that any attempt at laboratory isolations or monitoring have been reported.

C. trachomatis is sensitive to tetracyclines and erythromycin *in vitro*[48 52]. The first reported trial of a tetracycline backed by laboratory investigation was by Oriel *et al.*[53]. Minocycline was used, in a dosage of 100 mg twice daily for 3 weeks. Chlamydial isolations were carried out pre- and post-treatment, and resolution of symptoms with failure to re-isolate *C. trachomatis* was recorded. Female consorts were also included in this study, which thus constitutes one of the few trials on the treatment of female chlamydial infections. *C. trachomatis* could not be re-isolated after treatment of these women with minocycline. Prentice *et al.*[54] went further with laboratory studies, and looked for ureaplasmas as well as chlamydiae in their patients. Minocycline was again used, and this study was placebo controlled. A 200 mg dose of minocycline was given initially, followed by 100 mg twice daily for 6 days. Follow-up at seven days showed 28.5% of the placebo group to be symptom and sign free. The disappearance of symptoms and signs in the minocycline treated group correlated well with failure to re-isolate *C. trachomatis,* but less well with failure to re-isolate ureaplasmas.

The differential response of *Chlamydia*-positive and *Chlamydia*-negative NGU to tetracycline (1 g 6-hourly oxytetracycline for 6 days) was reported by Handsfield *et al.*[55]. Recurrence (the data does not allow distinction of relapse from re-infection) was more common in the *Chlamydia*-negative group. This is at variance with the earlier findings of Oriel *et al.*[5]. These results could be explained by a differential effect of treatment on *C. trachomatis* or ureaplasmas, related to duration of therapy[56]. Bowie *et al.*[57] have used the differential response to antimicrobials in an attempt to elucidate the role of *C. trachomatis* or ureaplasmas in NGU. Using sulphisoxazole (predominantly antichlamydial), and streptomycin or spectinomycin, (predominantly antiureaplasmal), they produced evidence that patients with *Chlamydia*-positive NGU responded better to sulphisoxazole, whilst patients with ureaplasma-positive, *Chlamydia*-negative NGU responded better to spectinomycin or streptomycin. The efficacy of the empirical use of sulphonamide/streptomycin combinations may thus be explained, and evidence of a role for both ureaplasmas and *C. trachomatis* is presented. From the clinical viewpoint, this study adds further weight to the use of tetracycline or erythromycin, as both infecting agents are sensitive to these antibiotics. A study by Vaughan-Jackson *et al.*[58] on post-gonococcal urethritis (PGU) found *C. trachomatis* to be causally related to the urethritis, but not *U. urealyticum*.

The duration of tetracycline therapy is controversial. Bowie[59] states that prolonging tetracycline therapy beyond 7 days does not seem justifiable. This comment is based on a minocycline trial comparing two doses, and two durations of therapy. A dose of 100 mg of minocycline twice daily was not found to be superior to 100 mg once daily. Others would advocate that a minimum of 14 days treatment is required. Prolonging the course to 21 days, particularly with 6-hourly regimens of tetracycline implies an unwarranted faith in patient compliance. The use of preparations with a longer half-life than oxytetracycline, such as doxycycline or minocycline may, by decreasing dose frequency, increase patient compliance. Oriel and his co-workers[60] carried out a treatment study with either 250 mg of oxytetracycline 6-hourly, or 500 mg of erythromycin stearate 12-hourly, each for 14 days. Patients were further divided into *Chlamydia*-positive or *Chlamydia*-negative groups. No difference in response was found between either drug, or between *Chlamydia*-positive and *Chlamydia*-negative groups, and it was concluded that erythromycin stearate is a satisfactory alternative to the tetracyclines in the treatment of NGU. It is interesting to note that some 20% of *Chlamydia*-positive patients relapsed after therapy with either drug, in the absence of any history of re-exposure to infection. This finding is common to all the treatment studies reported, and the significance is uncertain.

For the future, one antibiotic currently under development may be of use in NGU. Rosamicin, a macrolide related to erythromycin, is active against *C. trachomatis in vitro*[61 62]. Animal work with this antibiotic indicates the possibility that penetration into the prostatic fluid may be good[63 64]. Clinical studies with this agent are obviously needed.

C. trachomatis has now been identified as a major cause of epididymitis in men under the age of 35 years[65]. The use of tetracyclines or erythromycin is thus appropriate in this disease.

Current views on the treatment of NGU may be summarised as follows. Oxytetracycline 500 mg 6-hourly for one week will eradicate *C.*

trachomatis, but empirical studies of non-chlamydial NGU indicate that a duration of therapy of two weeks is often advantageous, and this regimen is recommended unless facilities for *C. trachomatis* isolation are available. Erythromycin stearate 500 mg 12-hourly for two weeks is a satisfactory alternative in patients in whom tetracyclines are contra-indicated.

A follow-up period of four weeks after completing therapy is advised, although not easy to attain in practice. Female sexual contacts of men with NGU should certainly be examined, as many have infections with *C. trachomatis* (and, indeed, with other organisms). Many physicians advocate 'epidemiological' treatment of these women with a tetracycline or erythromycin. The value of this in preventing recurrence in men is undecided, but in view of the prevalence of chlamydial infection in these women epidemiological treatment appears to be highly desirable.

On the assumption that PGU is caused by the same organisms that are associated with NGU, tetracycline or erythromycin are indicated for therapy. Dose schedules should be as for the treatment of NGU.

So-called 'non-specific genital infection' in women has been less studied with regard to treatment than NGU in men, and is indeed clinically an ill-defined entity. As with men, the full spectrum of pathogens is not known. *C. trachomatis* is associated with cervical discontinuity and cervical exudate, but like the gonococcus, may be isolated from the clinically normal cervix. Rees *et al.*[67] were able to relate resolution of cervical disease with the disappearance of *C. trachomatis* following treatment with oxytetracycline or erythromycin (250 mg 6-hourly for 21 days in each case).

The aetiology of acute salpingitis is becoming clearer. Recently, Mardh *et al.*[68] described the isolation of *C. trachomatis* from tubal cultures from 6 out of 20 women with acute salpingitis. *Mycoplasma hominis,* but not *U. urealyticum* is probably also involved in the pathogenesis of this disease[69]. Other evidence suggests that polymicrobial infection, particularly involving anaerobes may be a cause of pelvic inflammatory disease[70]. These findings seem to indicate that when considering therapy, there is little point in using penicillins or aminoglycosides in the absence of *N. gonorrhoeae.* Even here, however, clinical findings are controversial, as in a recent trial[71] it was found that penicillin or ampicillin or tetracycline were equally effective in the 'blind' therapy of acute salpingitis.

If any rationalisation is to be considered in the therapy of acute salpingitis, it seems logical initially to exclude the gonococcus. In the absence of *N. gonorrhoeae,* treatment should then be directed against the probable causative organisms. In this group must be placed *C. trachomatis,* the mycoplasmas, and anaerobic organisms. Therefore, the use of oxytetracycline (500 mg 6-hourly for 14 days) plus metronidazole (400 mg 8-hourly) is indicated. Erythromycin stearate (500 mg 12-hourly) although inactive against *M. hominis* is an alternative to oxytetracycline.

Male contacts of women with salpingitis should be identified, examined – in order to exclude the gonococcus – and treated for NGU.

Non-specific vaginitis is also enigmatic in aetiology. The discharge may be associated with *Haemophilus vaginalis,* but whether this is the prime pathogen remains controversial. This organism is said to be sensitive to ampicillin, and 500 mg 6-hourly for 10–14 days may be effective[72]. Others claim that metronidazole is a better drug to use[73]. Sulphonamide pessaries are of no value in this condition.

Future needs are obviously centred on the evaluation of the aetiology of NSGI. Only when this is understood can rational therapy be contemplated.

References

1 Oriel, J. D. (1978). Genito-urinary medicine. *Br. J. Venereal Dis.,* **54,** 291

2 Willcox, R. R. (1977). How suitable are available pharmaceuticals for the treatment of STD? 1: Conditions presenting as genital discharges. *Br. J. Venereal Dis.,* **53,** 314

3 Willcox, R. R. (1977). How suitable are available pharmaceuticals for the treatment of STD? 2: Conditions presenting as sores or tumours. *Br. J. Venereal Dis.,* **53,** 340

4 Falkow, S., Elwell, L. P., de Graaf, J., Heffron, F. and Meyer, L. (1976). A possible model for the development of plasmid-mediated penicillin resistance in the gonococcus. In R. D. Catterall and C. S. Nicol (eds.) *Sexually Transmitted Diseases,* pp. 120–133. (London: Academic Press)

5 Oriel, J. D., Reeve, P., Wright, J. T. and Owen, J. (1976). Chlamydial infection of the male urethra. *Br. J. Venereal Dis.,* **52,** 46

6 Holmes, K. K., Handsfield, H. H., Wang, S.-P., Wentworth, B. B., Turck, M., Anderson, J. B. and Alexander, E. R. (1975). Etiology of non-gonococcal urethritis. *N. Engl. J. Med.,* **292,** 1199

7 Tramont, E. C. (1976). Persistence of *Treponema pallidum* following penicillin G therapy. *J. Am. Med. Assoc.,* **236,** 2206

8 Mohr, J. A., Griffiths, W., Jackson, R., Saadah, H., Bird, P. and Riddle, J. (1976). Neurosyphilis and penicillin levels in cerebro-spinal fluid. *J. Am. Med. Assoc.,* **236, 2208**

9 Dees, J. E. and Colston, J. A. C. (1937). The use of sulphonamides in gonococci infections. Preliminary report. *J. Am. Med. Assoc.,* **108,** 1855

10 Olsen, G. A. and Lomholt, G. (1969). Gonorrhoea treated with a combination of probenecid and sodium penicillin G. *Br. J. Venereal Dis.,* **45,** 144

11 Groth, O. and Hallqvist, L. (1970). Oral ampicillin in gonorrhoea. *Br. J. Venereal Dis.,* **46,** 21

12 Bro-Jorgensen, A. and Jensen, T. (1971). Single-dose oral treatment of gonorrhoea in men and women, using ampicillin alone and combined with probenecid. *Br. J. Venereal Dis.,* **47,** 443

13 Eriksson, G. (1970). Oral ampicillin in uncomplicated gonorrhoea. 1: Treatment of

gonococcal urethritis in men. *Acta Dermatovenereologica (Stockholm),* **50,** 451

14 Eriksson, G. (1970). Oral ampicillin in uncomplicated gonorrhoea. 2: Results of treatment in women. *Acta Dermatovenereologica (Stockholm),* **50,** 461

15 Kvale, P. A., Keys, T. F., Johnson, D. W. and Holmes, K. K. (1971). Single oral dose ampicillin probenecid treatment of gonorrhoea in the male. *J. Am. Med. Assoc.,* **215,** 1449

16 Willcox, R. R. (1972). Amoxycillin in the treatment of gonorrhoea. *Br. J. Venereal Dis.,* **48,** 504

17 Thin, R. N., Symonds, R. A. E., Shaw, E. J., Wong, J., Hopper, P. K. and Slocombe, B. (1977). A double blind trial of amoxycillin in the treatment of gonorrhoea. *Br. J. Venereal Dis.,* **53,** 118

18 Price, J. D. and Fluker, J. L. (1975). Amoxycillin in the treatment of gonorrhoea. *Br. J. Venereal Dis.,* **51,** 398

19 Karney, W. W., Turck, M. and Holmes, K. K. (1974). Single oral dose therapy for uncomplicated gonorrhoea: Comparison of amoxycillin and ampicillin given with and without probenecid. *J. Infect. Dis.,* **129,** (Suppl.), 250

20 Willcox, R. R. (1976). Single oral dose of 1.5 g talampicin in the treatment of gonorrhoea. *Br. J. Venereal Dis.,* **52,** 184

21 Kaufman, R. E., Johnson, R. E., Jaffe, H. W., Thornsberry, C., Reynolds, G. H. and Weisner, P. J. (1976). National gonorrhoea monitoring study. Treatment results. *N. Engl. J. Med.,* **294,** 1

22 Phillips, I. (1976). β-lactamase-producing penicillin-resistant gonococcus. *Lancet,* **2,** 656

23 Ashford, W. A., Golash, R. G. and Hemming, V. G. (1976). Penicillinase-producing *N. gonorrhoeae. Lancet,* **2,** 657

24 Baron, E. S., Saz, A. K., Kopecko, D. J. and Wohlhieter, J. A. (1977). Transfer of plasmid-borne β-lactamase in *N. gonorrhoeae. Antimicrob. Agents Chemother.,* **12,** 270

25 Keys, T. F., Haverson, L. W., and Clarke, E. J. (1969). Single dose treatment of gonorrhoea with selected antimicrobial agents. *J. Am. Med. Assoc.,* **210,** 857

26 Willcox, R. R. (1971). Treatment of gonorrhoea with two oral doses of antibiotics. *Brit. J. Venereal Dis.,* **47,** 31

27 Arya, O. P., Rees, E., Percival, A., Alergant, C. D., Annels, E. H. and Turner, G. C. (1978). Epidemiology and treatment of gonorrhoea caused by penicillinase-producing strains in Liverpool. *Br. J. Venereal Dis.,* **54,** 28

28 Fowler, W., Rahim, G. and Brown, J. D. (1978). Clinical experience in the use of cefuroxime in gonorrhoea. *Br. J. Venereal Dis.,* **54,** 44

29 Xeri, L. and Orsolini, P. (1978). *In vitro* activity of cefuroxime against *T. pallidum. J. Antimicrob. Chemother.,* **4,** 189

30 Garrod, L. P. and Waterworth, P. M. (1968). Action of three drug combinations on gonococci. *Br. J. Venereal Dis.,* **44,** 75

31 Karney, W. W., Pedersen, A. H. B., Nelson, M., Adams, H., Pfeiffer, R. T. and Holmes, K. K. (1977). Spectinomycin versus tetracycline for the treatment of gonorrhoea. *N. Engl. J. Med.,* **296,** 889

32 Porter, I. A. and Rutherford, H. W. (1977). Treatment of uncomplicated gonorrhoea with spectinomycin hydrochloride. *Br. J. Venereal Dis.,* **53,** 115

33 Reyn, A., Schmidt, H., Trier, M. and Bentzon, M. W. (1973). Spectinomycin hydrochloride in the treatment of gonorrhoea: observation of resistant strains of *N. gonorrhoeae. Br. J. Venereal Dis.,* **49,** 54

34 Thornsberry, C., Jaffe, H., Brown, S. T., Edwards, T., Biddle, J. W. and

Thompson, S. E. (1973). Spectinomycin-resistant *N. gonorrhoeae. J. Am. Med. Assoc.*, **237**, 2405

35 Brown, S. T., Pedersen, A. H. R. and Holmes, K. K. (1977). Comparison of erythromycin base and estolate in gonococcal urethritis. *J. Am. Med. Soc.*, **238**, 1371

36 Sanders, C. C. and Sanders, W. E. (1977). *In vitro* activity of rosamicin against *Neisseria* and *Haemophilus,* including penicillinase-producing strains. *Antimicrob. Agents Chemother.*, **12**, 293

37 Masterton, G. and Schofield, C. B. S. (1976). Minocycline hydrochloride as a single-dose oral treatment of uncomplicated gonorrhoea in men. *Br. J. Venereal Dis.*, **52**, 43

38 Parriser, H. and Marino, A. F. (1970). One capsule treatment of gonorrhoea with minocycline. *Antimicrob. Agents Chemother.*, **5**, 211

39 Shahidullah, M. (1975). Single dose treatment of uncomplicated gonorrhoea in males with minocycline. *Br. J. Venereal Dis.*, **51**, 97

40 Willcox, R. R., (1963). Treatment of acute gonorrhoea with single injections of chloromycetin succinate. *Br. J. Venereal Dis.*, **39**, 160

41 Siboulet, A. (1972). Results of the minute treatment of gonorrhoea in 26 339 cases. *Postgrad. Med. J.*, **48** (Suppl. I), 63

42 Csonka, G. W. and Knight, G. T. (1967). Therapeutic trial of trimethoprim as a potentiator of sulphonamide in gonorrhoea. *Br. J. Venereal Dis.*, **43**, 161

43 Svinland, H. B. (1973). Treatment of gonorrhoea with sulphamethoxazole-trimethoprim. *Br. J. Venereal Dis.*, **49**, 50

44 Cobbold, R. J. C., Morrison, G. D. and Willcox, R. R. (1968). Treatment of gonorrhoea with single oral doses of rifampicin. *Br. Med. J.*, **2**, 681

45 Harkness, A. H. (1950). *Non-gonococcal Urethritis.* (Edinburgh: Livingstone)

46 Holmes, K. K., Johnson, D. W. and Floyd, T. M. (1967). Studies of Venereal Diseases. 3: Double-blind comparison of tetracycline hydrochloride and placebo in the treatment of non-gonococcal urethritis. *J. Am. Med. Assoc.*, **202**, 474

47 Willcox, R. R. (1972). "Triple tetracycline" in the treatment of non-gonococcal urethritis in males. *Br. J. Venereal Dis.*, **48**, 137

48 Ridgway, G. L., Owen, J. M. and Oriel, J. D. (1976). A method for testing the antibiotic susceptibility of *C. trachomatis* in a cell culture system. *J. Antimicrob. Chemother.*, **2**, 77

49 Treharne, J. D., Darougar, S., Jones, B. R. and Squires, S. (1977). Susceptibility of chlamydiae to chemotherapeutic agents. In D. Hobson and K. K. Holmes (eds.) *Non-gonococcal Urethritis and Related Infections,* pp. 214–222. (Washington DC: American Society for Microbiology)

50 Keshishyan, H., Hanna, L. and Jawetz, E. (1973). Emergence of Rifampicin-resistance in *C. trachomatis. Nature,* **244**, 173

51 Simopoulos, J. C. H. (1977). Tetracycline treatment for non-specific urethritis. *Br. J. Venereal Dis.*, **53**, 230

52 Ridgway, G. L., Owen, J. M. and Oriel, J. D., (1978). The antimicrobial susceptibility of *C. trachomatis* in cell culture. *Br. J. Venereal Dis.*, **54**, 103

53 Oriel, J. D., Reeve, P. and Nicol, C. S. (1975). Minocycline in the treatment of non-gonococcal urethritis. *J. Am. Venereal Dis. Assoc.*, **2**, 17

54 Prentice, M. J., Taylor-Robinson, D. and Csonka, G. W. (1976). Non-specific urethritis. A placebo controlled trial of minocycline in conjunction with laboratory investigations. *Br. J. Venereal Dis.*, **52**, 269

55 Handsfield, H. H., Alexander, E. R., Wang, S-P., Pedersen, A. H. and Holmes, K. K. (1976). Differences in therapeutic response of *Chlamydia*-positive and

Chlamydia-negative forms of non-gonococcal urethritis. *J. Am. Venereal Dis. Assoc.*, **2**, 5

56 Spaepen, M. S., Kundsin, R. B. and Horne, H. W. (1977). Tetracycline-resistant T-mycoplasmas from patients with a history of reproductive failure. *Antimicrob. Agents and Chemother.*, **9**, 1012

57 Bowie, W. R., Floyd, J. F., Miller, Y., Alexander, E. R., Holmes, J. and Holmes, K. K. (1976). Differential response of chlamydial and ureaplasma-associated urethritis to sulphafurazole (sulphisoxazole) and aminocyclitols. *Lancet*, **2**, 1276

58 Vaughan-Jackson, J. D., Dunlop, E. M. C., Darougar, S., Treharne, J. D. and Taylor-Robinson, D. (1977). Urethritis due to *C. trachomatis*. *Br. J. Venereal Dis.*, **53**, 180

59 Bowie, W. R. (1978). Etiology and treatment of non-gonococcal urethritis. *Sexually Transmitted Diseases*, **5**, 27

60 Oriel, J. D., Ridgway, G. L. and Tchamouroff, S. (1978). Comparison of erythromycin stearate and oxytetracycline in the treatment of non-gonococcal urethritis. *Scot. J. Med.*, **22**, 375

61 Ridgway, G. L. (1978). Unpublished data

62 Smith, T. F. and Washton, H. E. (1978). *In vitro* susceptibility of 30 strains of *C. trachomatis* to rosamicin. *Antimicrob. Agents Chemother.*, **14**, 493

63 Hoyme, U., Braumueller, A. and Madsen, P. O. (1977). Rosamicin in urethral and vaginal secretion and tissues in dogs. *Antimicrob. Agents Chemother.*, **12**, 237

64 Braumueller, A., Hoyme, U. and Madsen, P. O. (1977). Rosamicin:- a new drug for the treatment of bacterial prostatitis. *Antimicrob. Agents Chemother.*, **12**, 240

65 Berger, R. E., Alexander, E. R., Monda, G. D., Andsell, J., McCormick, G. and Holmes, K. K. (1978). *Chlamydia trachomatis* as a cause of 'idiopathic' epididymitis. *N. Engl. J. Med.*, **298**, 301

66 Oriel, J. D., Johnson, A. L., Barlow, D., Thomas, B. J., Nayyar, K. and Reeve, P. (1978). Infection of the uterine cervix with *C. trachomatis*. *J. Infect. Dis.*, **137**, 443

67 Rees, E., Tait, A., Hobson, D. and Johnson, F. W. A. (1977). *Chlamydia* in relation to cervical infection and pelvic inflammatory disease. In D. Hobson and K. K. Holmes (eds.) *Non-gonococcal Urethritis and Related Infections*, pp. 67–76. (Washington DC: American Society for Microbiology)

68 Mardh, P. A., Ripa, T., Svensson, L. and Westrom, L. (1977). *Chlamydia trachomatis* infection in patients with acute salpingitis. *N. Engl. J. Med.*, **296**, 1377

69 Mardh, P. A. and Westrom, L. (1970). Tubal and cervical culture in acute salpingitis with special reference to *Mycoplasma hominis* and T-strain mycoplasmas. *Br. J. Venereal Dis.*, **46**, 179

70 Eschenbach, D. A., Buchanan, T. M., Pollock, H. M., Forsyth, P. S., Alexander, E. R., Lin, J-S., Wang, S-P., Wentworth, B. B., McCormack, W. M. and Holmes, K. K. (1975). Polymicrobial aetiology of acute pelvic inflammatory disease. *N. Engl. J. Med.*, **293**, 166

71 Cunningham, F. G., Hauth, J. C., Strong, J. D., Herbert, W. N. P., Gilstrap, L. C., Wilson, R. H. and Kappus, S. S. (1977). Evaluation of tetracycline or penicillin and ampicillin for the treatment of acute pelvic inflammatory disease. *N. Engl. J. Med.*, **296**, 380

72 Rein, M. F. and Chapel, T. A. (1975). Trichomoniasis, Candidiasis, and the minor venereal diseases. *Clin. Obstet. Gynaecol.*, **18**, 73

73 Pheiffer, T. A., Forsyth, P. S., Durfee, M. A., Pollock, H. M. and Holmes, K. K. (1978). Nonspecific vaginitis: Role of *Haemophilis vaginalis* and treatment with metronidazole. *N. Engl. J. Med.*, **298**, 1429

6

Combinations of antibacterial drugs

N. A. Simmons

A few years ago I carried out a survey in a hospital in which I was then working and found that sufficient antibiotics were being dispensed by the pharmacy to maintain half of the patients in the hospital on antibiotics for the duration of their stay. However, on closer inspection it was apparent that fewer patients were receiving several antibacterial drugs and occasionally as many as three simultaneously. The reasons for the treatment were not always sound and combinations were sometimes given on the basis that two antibiotics were bound to be better than one. Similarly, the Lancet recently estimated that as many as one fifth of patients in hospital with infections receive two or more antibacterial agents concurrently[1]. The value of commercial preparations of fixed combinations of drugs is suspect[2] and in the past the sale of some combinations has been banned in the United States by the Food and Drug Administration[3]. Nevertheless, in Great Britain *MIMS* (the *Monthly Index of Medical Specialities*) lists in its sections on antibiotics, sulphonamides and antibacterials no fewer than 11 commercially available mixtures of antibacterial agents and, presumably, the pharmaceutical companies are not in the habit of producing preparations for which there is no demand.

In hospital antibiotics are often first prescribed by the doctors with the least experience who are more likely to be subject to criticism for ordering one test or one drug too few rather than one too many. In the circumstances it is not surprising that an antibiotic mixture may be given without a logical medical indication. That said, however, there are circumstances in which the administration of more than one antimicrobial agent may be quite justifiable.

The main reasons for the use of combinations of antibacterial agents may be summarized as follows:

157

(a) To achieve an additive or synergistic effect against a single organism. One of two objectives may be fulfilled by this. An organism may be successfully eradicated which cannot be eliminated by a single drug. Alternatively smaller amounts of each agent may be prescribed and dose-related toxic effects may be reduced;

(b) the prevention of the emergence of resistant organisms;

(c) the treatment of an infection due to two or more organisms which are not equally susceptible to a single agent;

(d) the early treatment of a serious infection before a bacteriological diagnosis can be made, the causative organisms isolated and their antibiotic susceptibilities determined.

Each of these reasons will be examined in turn.

EFFECTS OF COMBINATIONS

When two antibacterial agents act simultaneously upon a uniform microbial population the result may be addition, synergism, antagonism or indifference. At first sight these terms are easy to define, addition being said to be the result when the effect of the combination equals the sum of the antibacterial effects of its components, synergism when it exceeds that sum, antagonism when the effect of the combination is less than the most active component acting alone, and indifference when the activity of each component is unaffected by the presence of the other drug.

Unfortunately these definitions are imprecise since the criterion by which the activity of a drug or drug combination is measured must itself be defined and may be a source of confusion and controversy.

Should it be measured *in vivo* or *in vitro*? A variety of laboratory tests have been devised to demonstrate *in vitro* activity, whilst the *in vivo* activity has been measured in both animals and man. Jawetz and Gunnison (1952)[4] introduced an essential clinical element into their definition of synergism which they said was "a large increase in the rate of early bactericidal action and the rate of cure of infections beyond that obtainable by the simple additive effects of the agents". Similarly, they defined antagonism as "a large decrease in the rate of early bactericidal action and a reduction in the rate of cure of infections below that observed with the single more active drug." Twenty-seven years have passed since these definitions were published, but few antibiotic combinations can be said to have fulfilled these criteria. *In vitro* tests other than the demonstration of early bactericidal action or the lack of it are frequently employed because they are easier to perform and the correlation of *in vitro* tests with cure rates is not often demonstrated.

It is now more common for synergism to be defined purely in terms of the results of an *in vitro* test which, it is hoped, will predict the therapeutic value of a drug combination. One such test is the 'half chessboard' test[5] in which the activity against a given organism of a number of antibiotics added to broth in fixed concentrations singly and in every possible combination of two is determined. Both bacteristatic and bactericidal effects may be observed. A quantitative test is the chessboard titration in which tubes of liquid media are arranged in a square with the concentration of one drug decreasing from left to right and the other from top to bottom. In this way the 'chessboard' is made up of tubes which contain every possible combination of each of of the concentrations of the two agents. The tubes are inoculated and incubated and bacteristasis is shown by the absence of turbidity and bacterial killing by subculture. In this test synergism is usually defined as a combined effect at least four times as great as that of the more effective drug acting on its own. Alternatively, if the minimal inhibitory concentration (MIC) of each drug in the presence of the other is plotted on a graph (isobologram) in which the concentrations of the drugs are the axes, a line called an isobol is obtained (Figure 1). Characteristically a straight diagonal line across the graph represents addition, a line curved towards the lower concentrations indicates synergism and one bowed in the opposite direction indicates antagonism.

A method for quantifying the results of this test has been devised using what are called fractional inhibitory concentrations (FICs)[6]. The FIC is the MIC of one drug in the presence of the other, expressed as the fraction in decimal terms of its MIC when used alone. The FIC index is the sum of the FIC values of the two drugs when used in the best combination. Synergism is present when the index is less than 1.0, but it is customary to define it in terms of a lower figure; the lower the index the greater the synergism.

Whether an isobologram or FIC index or both are used to demonstrate the result, the chessboard test simply demonstrates the antibacterial effects after a fixed interval of time. It does not show the rate at which bacteria are killed. This can be demonstrated only by conventional killing curves in which the number of viable organisms in broth cultures containing the antibiotics under test, alone or in combination, are compared at regular intervals with each other and with a control culture which contains no drug. This method may be simplified and automated by measuring changes in the opacity of the broth culture, but growth inhibition and not killing are measured in this way.

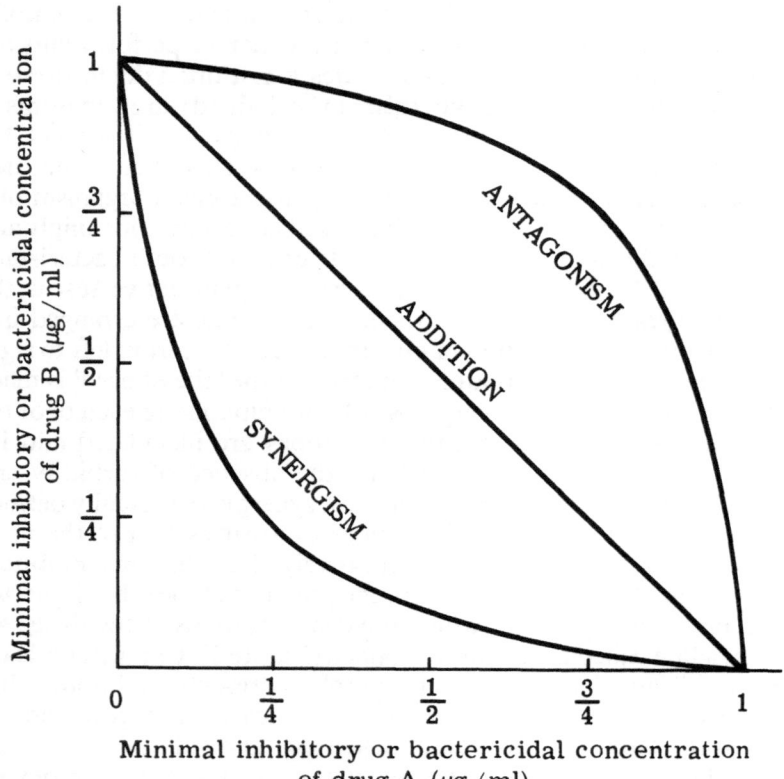

Figure 1 Isobologram. Isobols showing antagonism, addition and synergism

Tests using liquid media are time consuming and inconvenient and in diagnostic laboratories methods using solid media are more commonly employed. Conventional disc sensitivity tests may be done and drug interactions demonstrated in the area between two adjacent discs each of which contains one of the agents under investigation. Synergism may be expressed by enhanced inhibition in this area and antagonism by the flattening of that side of a zone of inhibition closest to the second disc. Alternatively the size of the zone of inhibition produced by a disc containing one drug on the surface of agar into which the other is incorporated may be compared with that on antibiotic free agar[7]. More commonly strips of blotting paper containing the antibiotics are used instead of discs. They are set at right angles to each other on the surface of a culture plate. If zones of inhibition which run parallel to each strip are reduced where both antibiotics are present in the angle where the strips touch, then this indicates antagonism. If the inhibition of growth is increased in this zone it indicates synergism. With most of these methods on solid media bacteristatic activity is usually determined by direct observation but bactericidal effects can also be demonstrated by replica plating[8] or the cellophane transfer technique[9] [10].

It is difficult if not impossible to state which of the many tests will predict most accurately the therapeutic effect of a combination of drugs in man. Each test has its disadvantages. For example, the chessboard and other techniques are subject to criticism on the grounds that the concentration of a drug and its antibacterial activity do not bear a linear relationship to each other[4] [11]. Half of the minimal inhibitory concentration of a given drug may inhibit the growth of well over half the strain being tested and yet most tests depend upon the demonstration of 100% inhibition. Tests using a 50% kill or inhibition could produce quite different results. The results of a single test may be difficult to interpret. I have seen chessboard tests which showed a combination synergistic in one set of concentrations and antagonistic in another. The combination of streptomycin and chloramphenicol may be antagonistic during the first few hours of exposure and synergistic later. Comparisons of tests may show good correlation[12], but unfortunately this is not always the case. Nevertheless, the examination of the activity of a drug combination against a wide variety of strains may well demonstrate a trend and give an indication of those species of bacteria with which synergism or antagonism are to be expected. It is now recognised that in a particular situation it is not possible to predict the effect with certainty, and in those cases in which knowledge of it is important, tests should be done using the organism which is the cause of the infection.

The animal model
Although it would be impractical to do tests in animals to show the activity of every drug combination against every organism causing an infection, the evaluation of fixed combinations in the treatment of animal infections is customary. Quite apart from the demonstration of toxic effects, which would not be apparent in an *in vitro* system, animal studies are usually considered to provide a more realistic simulation of the effect in man. Increasing amounts of agents under test may be administered singly and in combination to determine the dose which allows the survival of half or 90% of the animals studied. While such tests may be of considerable value caution is necessary in their interpretation since the pharmacokinetics of drugs in man and animals may differ significantly. For example, the half-lives of trimethoprim and sulphamethoxazole are both about 10 h in man, but are about 1 h and 3 h respectively in the rhesus monkey[13], and 1 h and 6 h in the mouse[14].

There are other problems. The normal bacterial flora and the pathogenicity of a bacterial species may be quite different in man and animals so that an artificial set of circumstances is required to produce an animal infection with a small number of bacteria, such as the concomitant injection of gastric mucin. However, *in vivo* tests like *in vitro* tests may demonstrate a trend which justifies the regular use of a particular drug combination.

Predictive schemes

It would be quite impossible for tests of combined antibacterial activity to be done in every patient with an infection. For this reason attempts have been made to produce guides to the expected effects of drug combinations based on existing knowledge. Perhaps the best known of these is 'Jawetz's Law'[4]. This holds that two bacteristatic drugs exert no more than an additive effect, that two bactericidal drugs may exert a synergistic effect and that a bactericidal plus a bacteristatic drug may show antagonism, which might be due to the fact that many bactericidal antibiotics exert their action only on multiplying bacteria and that if a second drug prevents multiplication the organisms survive. Suggestions for the modification of the Jawetz scheme which is now undoubtedly out of date have been made by Manten and Meyerman-Wisse[15][16] and Garrod and Waterworth[10].

The latter authors suggested that antibacterial agents should be divided into five groups:

(a) bacteristatic drugs which regularly antagonise bactericidal agents. This group includes chloramphenicol and tetracycline;

(b) drugs bacteristatic in low concentrations and bactericidal in higher concentrations. This group may antagonise or reinforce the action of other bactericidal antibiotics. It includes erythromycin and novobiocin;

(c) bactericidal drugs antagonised by bacteristatic agents. Drugs in this group kill multiplying bacteria and thus have their action interfered with by bacteristatic antibiotics. The group includes the penicillins, cephalosporins and aminoglycosides (e.g. streptomycin, neomycin and gentamicin);

(d) bactericidal drugs which are not antagonised by bacteristatic agents. This group includes the polymyxins and bacitracin which kill resting cells;

(e) bacteristatic drugs which act too slowly to antagonise bactericidal agents. The group includes the sulphonamides and cycloserine.

According to this scheme pairs of antibiotics drawn from group (c) are most likely to succeed in producing a bactericidal combination although combinations drawn from groups (b) and (c) may be successful. More recently Mouton[17] produced a modified version of the scheme produced by Manten and Meyerman-Wisse. It is shown in Figure 2.

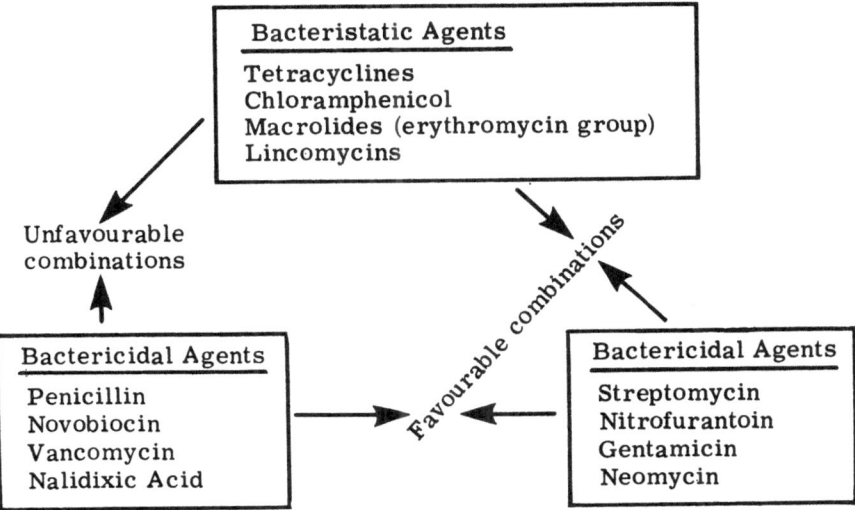

Figure 2   Mouton's scheme for predicting the affect of combinations of antibacterial drugs[17]

PREVENTION OF THE DEVELOPMENT OF RESISTANCE

The belief that the simultaneous administration of more than one antibacterial agent will prevent the emergence of resistant mutants is based largely on experience of the treatment of tuberculosis. The drug treatment of that disease is outside the scope of this Chapter, but the use of antituberculous drugs is employed here to illustrate the reasoning.

In a patient suffering from tuberculosis a few mycobacteria which have become resistant by spontaneous mutation to each of the anti-tuberculous drugs may be present. Therapy with a single drug selectively inhibits or kills susceptible bacteria allowing resistant mutants to survive and replace them. The early reports of treatment of tuberculosis with one drug such as streptomycin or isoniazid supported this theory. The concept of combined therapy was introduced on the basis that if one resistant mutant to drug A was present in 10^5 bacilli and one resistant mutant to drug B in 10^6 then the theoretical possibility of a mutant appearing which was resistant to both drugs was 1 in 10^{11}. For this reason it is normal practice for two or three antituberculous drugs to be administered simultaneously.

Unfortunately, although the practice is partially effective it does not completely prevent the emergence of resistant organisms and a variety of explanations have been offered for its failure to do so. First there is the problem of compliance; drugs may be prescribed, but they may not be taken by the patient. Secondly, when they are taken they may not reach the site of infection in an effective concentration. Thirdly, although the mycobacteria may be exposed to two drugs they may already be resistant to one of them. Thus combination therapy may be illusory in many cases, the reality being that organisms are being exposed to only one effective drug. Whatever the reason, when patients are subjected to multiple chemotherapy, mycobacteria resistant to one, two or even three agents may appear, albeit more slowly than in patients subjected to monotherapy.

Lacey[18] pointed out that it has never been established that combination chemotherapy succeeds in treating infections caused by *M. tuberculosis* by the suppression of the proliferation of resistant mutants. He felt that it was possible that the 'optimal' effect was produced in other ways possibly specific for this pathogen. Moreover, Hamilton-Miller and Brumfitt[19] have drawn attention to the fact that none of the many combinations used in the treatment of tuberculosis has been investigated for mutually potentiating effects, i.e. synergism. It is salutary to learn that in the disease in which combination therapy has been most carefully studied, wide gaps in our knowledge still exist.

Evidence that treatment of infections, other than tuberculosis, with combinations of antibiotics prevents the emergence of resistant mutants is surprisingly scanty. Kaipainen[20] showed that combinations of dihydrostreptomycin and tetracyclines (which are potentially antagonistic) could prevent the emergence of resistance.

Organisms exposed *in vitro* to trimethoprim alone develop a higher degree of resistance to this drug than they do when they are exposed to a mixture of trimethoprim and sulphamethoxazole, the components of co-trimoxazole, provided they are sensitive to both drugs[21]. However, *in vivo* a large number of organisms exposed to co-trimoxazole are resistant to sulphonamide and this has not led to the emergence of an appreciable number of trimethoprim resistant strains. In 1977 a survey of urinary pathogens in Birmingham, Bristol, Dublin and London showed that only 3% of 788 strains of *E. coli* isolated from patients with urinary tract infections were resistant to trimethroprim[22]. Of course, it could be argued that the number might have been greater had trimethoprim been marketed alone.

Combinations of subinhibitory concentrations of nalidixic acid and rifampicin have been shown to suppress the emergence of mutants resistant to each agent[23] and trimethoprim with rifampicin has also been shown to prevent the emergence of rifampicin resistant organisms[24].

It should be appreciated that the explanatory theory for the suppression of resistant organisms by antibiotic combinations applies only to those produced by mutation. It does not necessarily apply to organisms which become resistant by the acquisition of transferable R factors.

TREATMENT OF INFECTIONS CAUSED BY MORE THAN ONE ORGANISM

An infection caused by organisms which do not share a common antibiotic susceptibility is commonly cited as an indication for combined antimicrobial chemotherapy. However, those working in diagnostic bacteriology laboratories will be aware of the practical difficulties that often arise in making such a diagnosis. Many of the sites in which multiple infections occur are exposed to the patient's environment and the isolation of more than one organism on culture is not proof that they all are responsible for an infection. Cultures of material or swabs from lesions such as varicose ulcers or pressure sores more often than not grow several organisms, for most of which systemic chemotherapy is definitely not indicated. It is my belief that, in practice, cultures taken from this type of lesion may lead to worse rather than better treatment since subsequent treatment may be based on a mutual misunderstanding. The clinician believes that the microbiologists will report antibiotic sensitivities only if they believe the organisms isolated to be pathogenic. However, the differentiation between real pathogens, potential pathogens and commensals on the basis of the results of bacterial culture may be impossible. To be 'on the safe side' the laboratory reports what it finds – the organisms isolated and their sensitivity patterns – on the assumption that the doctor at the bedside will order antibiotics only if there are clinical indications for their prescription. Thus the stage is set for the needless administration of one or more drugs.

A similar situation may arise when specimens for culture are taken from sites such as ileostomies or colostomies when the organisms isolated simply represent the intestinal flora. In these situations it may be better to dispense with bacteriological cultures and base treatment, if clinically indicated, upon experience of clinical results. In this respect there is some evidence to suggest that treatment in the form of metronidazole directed specifically against non-sporing anaerobes may often be effective.

It could be argued that the treatment of infected postoperative abdominal wounds should always include metronidazole or another agent active against *Bacteroides* spp. and other Gram-negative anaerobes. Leigh *et al.*[25] recovered *Bacteroides fragilis* from 90% of wound infections after appendicectomy, but it used to be widely believed that such infections were usually caused by the Enterobacteriaceae or *Streptococcus faecalis* and it is only in recent years that the importance of the non-sporing anaerobes in abdominal sepsis has been widely recognised. That recognition is probably due to the more widespread use of improved laboratory methods. Indeed the frequency with which these organisms are isolated from infected abdominal wounds is probably a better indication of the quality of the specimens, the care taken in their collection and the culture techniques employed in the laboratory than of the presence of the organisms at the site of infection.

Although metronidazole is active against some strains of *Campylobacter jejuni* which are microaerophilic it is not active against other microaerophilic or aerobic organisms. Therefore when Enterobacteriaceae are also present, as they often are, metronidazole is usually given in combination with another antibiotic such as ampicillin or gentamicin. It has been suggested that *Bacteroides* spp. may have an adverse affect on leukocyte activity[26] and this has lent weight to the argument that an antibiotic active against them should be given whenever a mixed infection is suspected. On the other hand, Anderson[27] showed that R factor transfer is inhibited *in vitro* by dense suspensions of *B. fragilis* and he contended that suppression of anaerobes might increase the population of R factor carrying organisms and the frequency of R factor transfer and therefore the number of resistant organisms.

Salem, Jackson and McFadzean[28] showed that the action of metronidazole against *B. fragilis* was generally indifferent to the presence of other agents; *in vitro* it was potentiated slightly by sub-inhibitory concentrations of spiramycin, rifampicin, clindamycin and tetracycline and to a greater degree by nalidixic acid, but it did not interfere with the activity of 14 antibacterial agents against a variety of aerobes and facultative anaerobes. The 14 agents were ampicillin, cephalexin, chloramphenicol, co-trimoxazole, erythromycin, fusidic acid, gentamicin, nalidixic acid, neomycin, nitrofurantoin, novobiocin, rifampicin, spiramycin I and tetracycline. *In vivo* the CD_{50} values of 5 drugs (novobiocin, cephalexin, tetracycline, spiramycin I and fusidic acid) against *Staph. aureus*, and of 5 other drugs (ampicillin, chloramphenicol, rifampicin, nalidixic acid and co-trimoxazole) against an *E. coli* infection were not significantly affected by the simultaneous administration of metronidazole. Therefore, there seem to be no grounds for the limitation of the use of this drug on the basis of adverse reactions with other antibacterial agents.

Another drug active against anaerobes as well as Gram-positive organisms including *Staph. aureus* is clindamycin. In Britain it fell from favour with the advent of metronidazole and reports of the side effect of pseudomembranous colitis undoubtedly contributed to its loss of popularity. Killing curves used to demonstrate the combined effects of clindamycin and gentamicin, and of clindamycin and kanamycin revealed no evidence of antagonism with strains of *Staph. aureus, E. coli* and *Proteus mirabilis* and synergism with *B. fragilis*[29]. Chessboard tests of the combination of clindamycin and gentamicin showed it to be synergistic against many strains of *Staph. aureus, Str. pneumoniae, Str. pyogenes, Bacteroides* spp. and *Ps. aeruginosa*[30]. Although the concentrations required to demonstrate synergism were not readily obtainable *in vivo*, antagonism was never observed. In contrast, using a similar technique, Snyder *et al.*[31] showed the same combination to be antagonistic against *Str. mutans*, and Meers[32], using a different technique, showed it to be antagonistic against a strain of *Staph. aureus*. Meers also showed the combination of clindamycin and ampicillin to be antagonistic with the same organisms. The difficulties in the application of data acquired from *in vitro* tests to *in vivo* situations could not be more clearly demonstrated.

SERIOUS INFECTIONS

When a patient has a serious infection any delay in the institution of treatment may be critical and, therefore, it may have to be instituted before the results of bacteriological investigations are available. When there is no clue as to the nature of the infecting organism, which if allowed to multiply unchecked will lead to rapid deterioration in the condition of the patient, a combination of antimicrobial drugs may be given which has a spectrum of activity wide enough to cover the majority of potential pathogens. There are those who are prepared to select a combination whose action against some organisms may well be antagonistic; certainly, the administration of it may result in the multiplication (in the environment or in the patient) of resistant opportunistic micro-organisms and thereby cause infections which are even more difficult to treat, for no antibiotic combination can kill all of the organisms all of the time. Nevertheless, in exceptional circumstances these disadvantages may have to be accepted for the sake of the institution of early effective treatment. Diseases in which this situation may arise include leukaemia and meningitis.

Leukaemia

Neutropenia is a major factor predisposing to infection in patients with malignant disease and it is particularly liable to occur in acute leukaemia in which therapy inevitably results in bone marrow suppression. In this respect the treatment of myeloblastic leukaemia is more hazardous as the drugs employed are more likely to produce neutropenia than anti-lymphoblastic leukaemia therapy. The incidence of infection rises steeply when neutrophil counts fall below 1×10^9 per l. Susceptibility to infection is also increased by reduction in the numbers of monocytes and by the probable functional incompetence of both monocytes and the few neutrophils that are available in acute myeloblastic leukeamia. Impaired immunoglobulin synthesis is a factor of major importance in chronic lymphocytic leukaemia.

Although fungal and viral infections may occur bacteria are incriminated far more frequently and in most reports the Gram-negative bacilli predominate; *E. coli, Klebsiella* spp., *Proteus* spp. and *Serratia* spp. are common, and infections with *Ps. aeruginosa* carry a particularly poor prognosis. For this reason antibiotics are often chosen not only because of the broadness of the spectrum of their antibacterial activity, but also because of the likelihood of their achieving a synergistic effect against this particular pathogen.

Every effort is made to reduce the infection risk during anti-leukaemic treatment by the employment of reverse barrier nursing or plastic isolators. Prophylactic measures usually include the administration of antibiotics. A popular regime consists of the oral administration of the non-absorbable antibiotics framycetin, colistin and nystatin ('FRACON') together with the topical applications of chlorhexidine to the skin, hair, ears, nose, throat, mouth and vagina. The Leukaemia Research Fund trial[33] showed that this reduced the frequency of infection and of deaths due to infection. Lately it has been claimed that a less costly regime ('NEOCON') employing neomycin instead of framycetin and omitting many of the topical chlorhexidine applications is more convenient and equally effective[34].

The use of systemic antimicrobials in prophylaxis is more controversial. These have included co-trimoxazole[35] and more recently in rotation cephalexin, chloramphenicol, ampicillin, clindamycin, cephalothin, colistin sulphomethate, gentamicin, amphotericin B and 5-fluorocytosine. Success has been claimed for these regimes, but the long term effect of them and particularly the rotational scheme upon the environment in terms of the production of resistant bacteria could be grim. Because of the small numbers of neutrophils and the impaired inflammatory response, infection may be exceedingly difficult to diagnose in these patients. Regular culture of urine, stool, throat, sputum, axilla and vagina may suggest the nature of the infecting organisms, but fever is inevitably regarded as the best indication of infection and, rightly or wrongly, when it occurs most clinicians, having taken specimens for bacteriological examination, will start treatment. Granulocyte infusions may be valuable[36], but the main weapon is an antibiotic combination. At one time or another it has been claimed that the following combinations have been as successful as any other in neutropenic patients; carbenicillin and cephalothin, carbenicillin and gentamicin, cephalothin and gentamicin (although this combination was found to be substantially more nephrotoxic than the other two, causing renal dysfunction in 12% of cases[37]), methicillin, carbenicillin, cephalothin, gentamicin and clindamycin[38], tobramycin and clindamycin[39] and tobramycin and cephalothin[40].

It is difficult to compare the results of treatment in different trials, but on first principles one should use as few antibiotics as possible in a combination and at this time the combination of carbenicillin and gentamicin is not an unreasonable choice, gentamicin alone having been shown to be not always effective in severe infections in neutropenic patients. The results of the trial of tobramycin with clindamycin[39] were also impressive.

Meningitis
The controversy between advocates and opponents of combination therapy is well illustrated in the case of meningitis. Excluding neonatal disease with which I shall deal separately, the vast majority of cases of meningitis are caused by three species of bacteria: *Haemophilus influenzae, Streptococcus pneumoniae* and *Neisseria meningitidis*. Provided the nature and sensitivity of the infecting organism is known, there is little dispute about the recommended treatment for sensitive strains; a sulphonamide such as sulphadiazine, sulphafurazole or sulphadimidine for meningococci, benzyl penicillin for pneumococci and chloramphenicol or ampicillin for *H. influenzae*. There is some dispute about the need to administer penicillin and ampicillin by the intrathecal as well as by a systemic route, the advocates stressing the advantages of a high concentration of active drug at the site of infection at an early stage, the opponents arguing that when the meninges are inflamed both drugs diffuse readily into the cerebrospinal fluid. For those who wish to give intrathecal injections the maximum recommended dose of benzyl penicillin is 3 mg (5000 units) for an infant and 6 mg (10 000 units) for an

older child or an adult, and of ampicillin between 5 and 8 mg for infants and between 10 and 40 mg for adults. Elsewhere I have deliberately refrained from discussing dosage, but I do so here because I have seen more than one case of massive intrathecal overdose which has led to cerebral irritation and death.

It is in discussions about the initial therapy for meningitis or therapy for meningitis of unknown aetiology that disputes arise over the desirability of combination therapy. In 1951 Jawetz *et al.*[41] reported that chloramphenicol antagonised the bactericidal action of penicillin on streptococci and *Klebsiella* spp. *in vitro*. In the same year Lepper and Dowling[42] reported that penicillin alone was superior to penicillin plus chloretetracycline in the treatment of pneumococcal meningitis. In their study 3 of 14 penicillin treated patients died (21%) compared with 11 of 14 patients treated with penicillin and chlortetracycline (79%). Both chloramphenicol and the tetracyclines are bacteristatic drugs which inhibit protein synthesis, but their binding sites differ. In 1967, Wallace *et al.*[43] studied the effect of combinations of penicillin and chloramphenicol on experimental canine pneumococcal meningitis. They found that chloramphenicol inhibited the bactericidal action of penicillin both *in vitro* and *in vivo*. In the latter situation, antagonism was most marked when chloramphenicol was administered before penicillin and the organisms were completely eradicated when both antibiotics were given for more than six hours. The authors concluded that significant clinical antagonism would occur only in patients exposed to broad spectrum bacteristatic antibiotics before the institution of penicillin therapy. One would not expect penicillin to antagonise the action of chloramphenicol on susceptible organisms and combinations of the two drugs have been used with success in studies of pneumococcal pneumonia[44 45].

Given this background two schools of thought have emerged. There are those who would treat meningitis initially with a combination of three drugs, penicillin, chloramphenicol and a sulphonamide[46], or two drugs, penicillin and chloramphenicol[47], and others who believe that as all three common bacterial species responsible for the disease are susceptible to chloramphenicol this drug may be used alone or alternatively ampicillin alone in large intravenous doses. The emergence of ampicillin resistant strains of *H. influenzae* has been a factor favouring the use of chloramphenicol.

As is commonly the case in disputes over combinations of antibacterial agents the argument may become heated and Christie[48] stated that in the treatment of pyogenic meningitis of unknown aetiology "to treat such patients with 3 or 4 drugs, as is sometimes done, reflects confusion of thought both as regards the nature of antimicrobial action and the bacteriology of meningitis".

My own view has changed in recent years. I used to be an advocate of triple therapy although I stressed the need to modify treatment by discontinuing unnecessary drugs when the results of investigations became available for I had seen more than one case in which meningococci had been persistently isolated from the cerebrospinal fluid of patients on triple therapy and had been eliminated only when the administration of chloramphenicol had been stopped. Now I prefer monotherapy with chloramphenicol.

Neonatal meningitis
Meningitis is a frequent complication of septicaemia in the newborn having a poor prognosis with high mortality and a high risk of residual neurological damage. Predisposing factors include prematurity, neurological defects, perinatal infection in the mother and premature rupture of the membranes. It is said to occur in about one in 2000 infants although in premature infants the incidence is nearly 8 times higher. Any organism may cause the disease in the newborn but Gram-negative bacilli, including *E. coli, Aerobacter* and *Klebsiella* spp., *Proteus* spp. and *Ps. aeruginosa*, are particularly common, and streptococci including those of Group B are also a significant cause. Because of the nature of the potentially infecting organisms, gentamicin is generally recommended, but to ensure that it reaches the CSF in an adequate concentration it must be given by the intrathecal or intraventricular as well as the systemic route. Since it is relatively inactive against streptococci it is usually combined with another drug which may be a cephalosporin or a penicillin such as ampicillin also given both systemically and intrathecally. The antibacterial effect of combinations of the β-lactam antibiotics (penicillins and cephalosporins) and aminoglycosides is discussed later.

Lorber[49] regards the management of neonatal meningitis as "the paediatric equivalent of open heart surgery" and believes that it should not be attempted in any but special centres. He considers the risk of early ineffective treatment as an overriding factor and therefore recommends treatment with a combination of chloramphenicol and gentamicin, both being administered by the systemic and intrathecal or intraventricular routes. The choice of this drug combination is open to question, since its effect might be expected to be antagonistic and the systemic administration alone of chloramphenicol should result in adequate CSF levels. Gentamicin with chloramphenicol was shown to be less effective in clearing bacteria from the CSF of rabbits with *Pr. mirabilis* meningitis than gentamicin alone[50]. Rahal[51] reviewed the reports of the effect of the combination and concluded that, whereas *in vitro* tests consistently demonstrated antagonism, the results of animal tests varied and no clinical evidence was available on the use of the combination in Gram-negative infections which supported or refuted the possibility of antagonism.

DISADVANTAGES OF COMBINATION THERAPY

(a) *Antagonism* – I have already discussed antagonism at length and examples were given in the section on meningitis. However, the work of Manten and Meyerman-Wisse[16] is worthy of special mention. In a systematic *in vitro* study using antibiotic discs and a replica plating technique they demonstrated antagonism with the pairs of drugs shown in Table 1. They graded the effect and some pairs were said to show only partial antagonism.

(b) *Adverse drug effects* – The number of adverse drug reactions increases with the number of drugs administered and antibiotics can be a major cause of them[52]. The need for the sulphamethoxazole component of co-trimoxazole has been questioned on the grounds that the majority of side effects appears to be due to it.

With some antibiotic pairs the toxic effects are enhanced. Mention has already been made of the high incidence of nephrotoxicity in patients given cephalothin and gentamicin[37], and the same enhanced toxic effect has been observed with the combination of colistin and cephalothin[53]. It has been suggested that additive hepatotoxic effects could occur with combinations of tetracyclines and erythromycin[54], although this seems unlikely to be a risk if erythromycin estolate is avoided.

(c) *Inactivation* – Carbenicillin may cause the physical inactivation of gentamicin[55], but if solutions of the two drugs are freshly prepared or administered separately the effect is unlikely to be of importance in the clinical situation except in the presence of severe impairment of renal function with delayed excretion and prolonged intervals between doses. Carbenicillin has also been shown to inactivate kanamycin, and gentamicin may also be inactivated slowly by high concentrations of ampicillin, penicillin, methicillin and cloxacillin[56], but the effect is unlikely to be of any clinical significance as the concentrations required are very much higher than the normal therapeutic level. Lynn[57] showed that precipitation occurred when solutions of benzyl penicillin, ampicillin, cloxacillin or flucloxacillin were mixed with a solution of polymyxin B, or a solution of ampicillin with colistin. Crystallisation occurred when solutions of penicillin "at intramuscular concentrations" were added to vials containing lincomycin hydrochloride.

Table 1   Pairs of antibacterial agents showing antagonism

Antagonism against Staph. aureus	*Antagonism against* Strept. faecalis
Penicillin + tetracycline	Penicillin + tetracycline
Penicillin + chloramphenicol	Penicillin + chloramphenicol
Penicillin + erythromycin	Penicillin + erythromycin
Tetracycline + neomycin*	
Tetracycline + bacitracin*	
Tetracycline + vancomycin	
Tetracycline + ristocetin	*Antagonism against* Salmonella *spp.*
Tetracycline + novobiocin	Streptomycin + tetracycline*
Chloramphenicol + neomycin	Streptomycin + chloramphenicol
Chloramphenicol + bacitracin	Tetracycline + chloramphenicol
Chloramphenicol + vancomycin	Tetracycline + neomycin*
Chloramphenicol + ristocetin	Chloramphenicol + neomycin*
Chloramphenicol + novobiocin	
Erythromycin + neomycin*	
Erythromycin + bacitracin*	
Erythromycin + vancomycin	
Erythromycin + ristocetin	
Erythromycin + novobiocin	
Novobiocin + vancomycin*	
Novobiocin + ristocetin*	

* = partial antagonism

Lynn concluded that solutions of these drugs for intramuscular injection should never be mixed in the syringe.

(d) *Difficulty in diagnosis* – If a patient with an infection is treated with several antibacterial drugs and fails to respond a difficult diagnostic problem may be set. Persistent fever may be due to one of the drugs or infection which in turn may be due to the fact that no effective drug has been given or due to antagonism of one potentially effective agent by another. Unfortunately, it is all too often the case that advice is sought only when difficulties of this nature arise.

(e) *Opportunistic infections* – No combination of drugs, however synergistic their action and however broad their spectrum, can be active against all potential pathogens. The administration of numerous drugs, particularly as a prophylactic measure, is most likely to result in the eventual multiplication of and infection with unusual opportunistic micro-organisms such as viruses or fungi.

(f) *Cost* – The unnecessary prescription of antibiotics is an expensive exercise. It has been calculated that amikacin is four times as expensive as pure gold. In my own hospital more than £7000 was spent in a ten month period on an antibiotic on which the results of *in vitro* sensitivity tests were never reported.

COMMENTS ON PARTICULAR COMBINATIONS

Co-trimoxazole

All cells require tetrahydrofolic (folinic) acid for purine synthesis. Tetrahydrofolic acid is generated from dihydrofolic (folic) acid, the action being catalysed by the enzyme dihydrofolic acid reductase. Man absorbs his folate pre-formed from food, but parasites, with rare exceptions, cannot do so and must synthesise folate using as a starting material para-aminobenzoic acid (PABA). The bacterial synthesis of folate is catalysed by the enzyme dihydrofolic acid synthetase and is inhibited by sulphomamides.

Trimethoprim is a diaminopyrimidine, compounds of which have as a general property the ability to inhibit the enzyme dihydrofolic acid reductase. Modification of the molecule can greatly increase the activity against the enzyme of one species whilst decreasing it against another. Trimethoprim, 2,4-diamino-5(3,4,5-trimethoxybenzyl)pyrimidine, has an affinity for the bacterial enzyme approximately 50 000 times greater than for the human enzyme. Furthermore, man unlike bacteria can also absorb pre-formed folinic acid thereby by-passing the action of the drug. Thus in bacteria sulphonamides and trimethoprim act sequentially on two steps in the same metabolic pathway. The result of this sequential blockade is that the two compounds produce a marked antimicrobial synergy[58].

In addition trimethoprim and sulphonamide acting alone are bacteristatic, but combinations of the two are frequently bactericidal. For these reasons when trimethoprim was first marketed in Britain in 1969 it was made available only as a mixture with sulphamethoxazole in a weight-to-weight ratio of 1 : 5 respectively under the official name co-trimoxazole. The mixture has a broad antibacterial spectrum which encompasses Gram-negative bacteria including *H. influenzae, E. coli, Salmonella, Shigella* and *Proteus* spp., and Gram-positive organisms including *Staph. aureus, Str. viridans* and *Str. faecalis.*

Sulphamethoxazole is one of the most active sulphonamides and was selected for the combination because of its pharmacokinetic properties which resemble those of trimethoprim in many respects. Both drugs are rapidly absorbed from the gut and 90% of each can be recovered from the urine, although in the case of sulphamethoxazole only about half the drug is excreted in an antibacterially active form. The plasma half-lives of both agents in man are about 10 hours, but there are pharmacokinetic discrepancies. The volume of distribution of trimethoprim which is concentrated in some tissues is slightly greater than the total body water, whereas sulphamethoxazole is apparently restricted to the extracellular fluid. As a consequence, a given dose of sulphamethoxazole results in a plasma level approximately four times greater than the level of trimethoprim achieved by taking the same amount of that drug and the administration of the drugs as co-trimoxazole results in a plasma concentration of sulphamethoxazole about twenty times that of trimethoprim. With the majority of organisms this ratio of concentrations produces the maximum *in vitro* synergistic effect[58], but there are notable exceptions such as *Brucella* and *Neisseria* spp. with which synergy is optimum when the concentration of trimethoprim exceeds that of sulphonamide. Furthermore, the different pattern of distribution of the two components in the tissues makes it likely that the optimal ratio is not always achieved at the site of infection or inside cells.

In vitro synergy has been observed even with some sulphonamide resistant organisms and this has been given as one reason for the refusal to release trimethoprim except in combination with a sulphonamide.

There is no doubt that co-trimoxazole has proved to be effective in the treatment of infections of the respiratory and urinary tract, but. trimethoprim alone has been shown to be at least as effective as co-trimoxazole in the treatment of urinary tract infections in domiciliary practice and bacteriuria of pregnancy[59]. A second reason given for the mandatory inclusion of a sulphonamide is that it might be expected to prevent or delay the emergence of resistant organisms. However, with the many sulphonamide resistant organisms now isolated, particularly from infections of the urinary tract, this argument is not applicable. At the present time there appears to be a perceptible swing towards the view that trimethoprim alone should be released as a preparation, a view reinforced by the observation that the majority of toxic reactions to co-trimoxazole appear to be due to the sulphonamide component.

It is ironic that at such a moment a new sulphonamide–trimethoprim mixture should make its commercial debut. In co-trimazine the sulphonamide component is sulphadiazine, chosen because it reaches the urine largely in an antibacterially active form. The use of co-trimazine is advocated only in the treatment of urinary tract infections; the recommended dose is less than co-trimoxazole, and the ratio of trimethoprim to sulphadiazine is 1 : 4.5. It remains to be seen whether this mixture has any advantage over co-trimoxazole. Even if it does, the extent of the comparative clinical trial required to demonstrate a statistically significant difference could be daunting.

Meanwhile a new diaminopyrimidine–sulphonamide mixture of tetroxoprim and sulphadiazine has appeared over the therapeutic horizon. Unless it is demonstrably more effective or cheaper than co-trimoxazole, an unlikely prospect at the present time, it will not constitute a significant therapeutic advance.

Polymyxins, sulphonamides and trimethoprim
There have been many reports of synergism between polymyxins and sulphonamides and polymyxins and trimethoprim against Gram-negative organisms. *Proteus* and *Serratia* spp. which are resistant to the polymyxins can be rendered sensitive to them by sulphonamide or trimethoprim and *in vitro* synergy has been demonstrated between a polymyxin, sulphonamide and trimethoprim acting together, a combination used successfully in clinical infections with *Pseudomonas* and *Proteus* spp. including endocarditis. The literature has been reviewed by Simmons[60] and Rahal[51]. Explanations for the synergistic effect include the suggestion that the sulphonamide allows greater penetration of the cell wall by the polymyxin allowing it more readily to reach the cell membrane where it exerts its effect, and sequential blockade, for polymyxins, like the other two components, inhibits a step in purine synthesis. Unfortunately, but characteristically, antagonism between a polymyxin and sulphonamide against *Ps. aeruginosa* has also been demonstrated.

Combinations of β-lactam antibiotics (penicillins, cephalosporins and cephamycins)
Two commercial preparations of fixed combinations of penicillins are marketed in Britain at the present time, 'Ampiclox' which contains ampicillin and cloxacillin, and 'Magnapen' which contains ampicillin and flucloxacillin. Both mixtures are intended for use in severe infections when the causative organisms are unknown, the cloxacillin or flucloxacillin component being included to cover the possible presence of penicillinase-producing staphylococci, and the ampicillin to broaden the antimicrobial spectrum to include Gram-negative organisms. I have

already commented in general on the value of preparations containing fixed amounts of antibacterial agents, but the manufacturer's suggested indication for their use in this case is only one of a possible three for the administration of combinations of β-lactam antibiotics.

A second might be a severe staphylococcal infection, for example pneumonia, for which the patient requires immediate treatment and it is not known whether or not the organism is a producer of penicillinase. In these circumstances most doctors using a penicillin would use only a β-lactamase resistant variety such as methicillin, cloxacillin or flucloxacillin, or a cephalosporin which would be active both against those staphylococci which produce penicillinase and against those which do not. However, there are doctors who would give benzyl penicillin as well as a penicillinase-stable compound[61], arguing that the former being a hundred or more times as active as the latter against staphylococci which do not produce penicillinase would constitute far more effective treatment for infections with them; although it would be ineffective against producers of penicillinase it would not adversely affect the action of the β-lactamase-stable compound against these organisms.

Theoretically a third indication for the administration of a combination of β-lactam antibiotics would be an attempt to achieve a synergistic effect against Gram-negative bacteria. In 1964[62-64] it was shown that methicillin and cloxacillin, which were themselves virtually inactive against Gram-negative organisms, enchanced the activity of ampicillin, benzyl penicillin, cephalosporin C, cephalothin and cephaloridine against some enterobacteria. It was shown that synergism was achieved by virtue of competitive inhibition by methicillin and cloxacillin of the β-lactamase produced by the Gram-negative organisms. The two antibiotics appeared to have a greater affinity for the enzyme and were not hydrolysed by it. This situation is the reverse of that which exists with staphylococci where the antibiotics with the poorest affinity for the bacterial enzyme are the least hydrolysed. Unfortunately, although synergism is clearly demonstrable *in vitro* with certain strains of Gram-negative bacteria, they are in a minority and the amounts of the drugs required to achieve synergism are so high that the phenomenon has few practical applications although combinations of these agents have been employed to treat infections of the urinary tract.

Marked *in vitro* synergism between oxacillin and ampicillin against enterococci has been described recently[65] and the combination was used successfully in the treatment of a patient with endocarditis. As the enterococci did not produce β-lactamase an explanation other than that given above should be sought for this effect.

An interesting recent development has been the discovery of naturally occurring substances, of which clavulanic acid is an example, which themselves have negligible antibacterial activity, but which in low concentrations inhibit β-lactamases and thus extend the range of activity of antibiotics destroyed by them.

Unfortunately combinations of penicillins and cephalosporins are occasionally antagonistic; although rare this has been seen with cloxacillin and ampicillin, and with carbenicillin and cephaloridine and the reason for it is a matter of controversy. One hypothesis is that the less active antagonist has a greater affinity for a site on the bacteria where the more active drug would be most effective. The more potent agent is therefore driven to a 'less sensitive' site. Another hypothesis is that as a result of mutation the less active component produces minor changes in the target enzyme of the more active drug.

Mecillinam

Mecillinam is an antibiotic similar to the penicillins which differs from them in some important respects. Other penicillins are derivatives of 6-aminopenicillanic acid; mecillinam is a derivative of amidinopenicillanic acid and has a different antibacterial spectrum. Mecillinam itself is not absorbed from the gastrointestinal tract, but its pivaloyloxymethyl ester, pivmecillinam, is absorbed and at present is the only marketed preparation. Pivmecillinam itself has no antibacterial activity, but it is rapidly hydrolysed during absorption liberating mecillinam.

Most penicillins are more active against Gram-positive than Gram-negative organisms, but with mecillinam the reverse is the case. Many Gram-negative organisms, with the exception of *Haemophilus* and *Neisseria* spp. are sensitive to low concentrations. The drug exhibits a high *in vitro* activity against strains of *E. coli, Klebsiella, Enterobacter, Citrobacter, Salmonella* and *Shigella* species, and *Pr. mirabilis* and *vulgaris. Pseudomonas* and *Bacteroides* spp. are resistant. There are technical difficulties in demonstrating *in vitro* sensitivity to this agent. The results are dependent on inoculum size and the osmolality and conductivity of the media employed. In media of high osmolality and conductivity the activity of the drug is considerably decreased. The MBC may be very much higher than the MIC. Although mecillinam interferes with the biosynthesis of the bacterial cell wall it has a mode of action on Gram-negative bacilli which differs from that of other β-lactam antibiotics. It binds only the second penicillin-binding protein in the envelope of *E. coli* (benzyl penicillin will bind up to eight proteins) resulting in the formation of large spherical cells. Consequently, it was thought that it might act synergistically with other β-lactam antibiotics and it has been shown to do so. Neu[66] demonstrated synergism with some isolates of the *Enterobacteriaceae*, provided they were resistant or only moderately sensitive to mecillinam, when mecillinam was combined with ampicillin, amoxycillin, cephalothin, cephamandole or cefoxitin. Synergism could not be demonstrated with strains highly sensitive to mecillinam when only MICS were considered, but it was demonstrated by the MBCs. Synergism between mecillinam and ampicillin has also been demonstrated *in vitro* against *H. influenzae*. Cloxacillin also exhibits a synergistic effect by inhibiting β-lactamase to which mecillinam is susceptible.

In vivo synergism between mecillinam and other β-lactam antibiotics has been demonstrated in protection studies in mouse[67] and in man[68] in the treatment of purulent exacerbations of chronic bronchitis and *Salmonella enteritidis* endocarditis[69].

Combinations of the β-lactam antibiotics and aminoglycosides
Streptococci are the commonest cause of endocarditis, *Str. viridans* being the variety most frequently incriminated, but others particularly those of Group D also being implicated. Those in Group D can be broadly classified into the enterococci including *Str. faecalis* and *Str. faecium* and the non-enterococcal species, *Str. bovis*.

The treatment of enterococcal endocarditis is probably the most firmly established indication for treatment with an antibiotic combination. For many years benzyl penicillin and streptomycin have been regarded as the standard therapy, but with the development of new β-lactam and aminoglycoside antibiotics, the possibility of finding an even more effective combination has been examined. The subject has been reviewed by Watt[70] and Rahal[51]. In 1950 Jawetz and Gunnison[71] reported that when *Str. faecalis* was exposed to penicillin, although there was an initial bactericidal effect, it was incomplete. The addition of streptomycin in a concentration that was ineffective on its own resulted in a more rapid and complete bactericidal effect. Subsequently the combination of penicillin and streptomycin was shown to be effective in the treatment of *Str. faecalis* endocarditis[72]. It has since been shown that enterococci fall into two groups; those that exhibit low-level resistance to streptomycin with an MIC of 25–100 μg/ml and those which are resistant to a much higher concentration with an MIC greater than 2000 μg/ml. Synergism between penicillin and streptomycin occurs only with the more sensitive enterococcal strains. Similarly, some (but fewer) strains of enterococci are highly resistant to kanamycin and with these synergism between penicillin and kanamycin cannot be demonstrated. In contrast, penicillin and gentamicin appear to have a synergistic action against all strains of enterococci, the MIC of the aminoglycoside being generally less than 50 μg/ml. There is, therefore, a strong argument in favour of making gentamicin the aminoglycoside component of the combination.

Is benzyl penicillin the best β-lactam component? Ampicillin and amoxycillin are more active against enterococci and combinations of each of these drugs with gentamicin have been shown to be synergistic and bactericidal with these organisms. *In vitro* the combination of amoxycillin and tobramycin has been shown to be as effective, but combinations of amoxycillin and either streptomycin or kanamycin are not synergistic against strains highly resistant to the aminoglycoside. The combination of amoxycillin and amikacin is not synergistic with strains highly resistant to kanamycin although they may appear relatively sensitive to amikacin itself. Other combinations usually showing synergism with enterococci *in vitro* include benzyl penicillin or ampicillin plus sissomicin or netilmicin; of the four possible combinations of these drugs penicillin and sissomicin appears to be the most active. The combination of cephalothin and streptomycin is synergistic against some enterococcal strains, but clinical results have been poor. In summary, enterococcal endocarditis is best treated with a combination of a penicillin and an aminoglycoside. The penicillin component may be benzyl penicillin with which we have the most experience, but the use of ampicillin or amoxycillin is fully justified. Of the aminoglycosides gentamicin is probably the best in practice, although streptomycin can be used provided that the organism causing the infection has been shown by laboratory tests not to have a high level of resistance to it.

Endocarditis caused by *Str. bovis* and *Str. viridans* may be treated by a penicillin alone. Amoxycillin and benzyl penicillin have similar activity and both compounds are slightly more active than ampicillin. In contrast to the situation with enterococci the MBCs of all three compounds for *Str. viridans* and *Str. bovis* are only slightly higher than the MICs. However, even with these organisms the rate at which killing takes place is enhanced by an aminoglycoside provided that the streptococci are not highly resistant to it. For this reason a good case can be made for using combination therapy in the treatment of endocarditis caused by non-enterococcal streptococci.

Organisms other than streptococci
Interactions between aminoglycosides and β-lactam antibiotics have been demonstrated with organisms other than streptococci and some examples are given in Table 2. Farrell, Wilks and Drasar[73] investigated the combined effect of three semi-synthetic penicillins, carbenicillin, azlocillin and mezlocillin and three aminoglycosides gentamicin, tobramycin and amikacin against 138 gentamicin resistant Gram-negative rods. They made a distinction between "*in vitro* synergy" and "useful synergy" the latter judged by obtainable serum levels. Potentially useful synergism was found between gentamicin and carbenicillin

with *Ps. aeruginosa, Proteus* spp., *Providencia* spp., *Acinetobacter* spp. and *Alkaligens* spp. Combinations of azlocillin and each of the aminoglycosides, and mezlocillin and gentamicin displayed synergism against *Ps. aeruginosa*.

Table 2 Results of some reports of interaction between penicillins and aminoglycosides

Antibiotic Combination		Organism	Synergism	Antagonism	Ref.
Penicillin	*Aminoglycosides*				
Ampicillin	Kanamycin		+	−	74
Ampicillin	Streptomycin	*Proteus mirabilis*	+	−	74
Ampicillin	Gentamicin*		+	−	74
Penicillin	Gentamicin		+	−	74
Ampicillin	Kanamycin*		+	+	74
Ampicillin	Streptomycin	Indole positive	−	−	74
Ampicillin	Gentamicin	*Proteus* spp.	+	+	74
Penicillin	Gentamicin		+	+	74
Carbenicillin	Gentamicin	*Ps aeruginosa*	+	−	90
Carbenicillin	Amikacin*		+	−	91
Carbenicillin	Gentamicin	*Serratia marcescens*	+	−	91
Carbenicillin	Tobramycin		+	−	91
Carbenicillin	Gentamicin		+	−	92
Carbenicillin	Tobramycin		+	−	92
Carbenicillin	Amikacin	*Staph. aureus*	+	−	92
Ticarcillin	Gentamicin		+	−	92
Ticarcillin	Tobramycin*		+	−	92
Ticarcillin	Amikacin		+	−	92

* = Most synergistic combination

It is unfortunate that combinations of β-lactam and aminoglycoside antibiotics are not universally synergistic and that antagonism has occasionally been demonstrated[74]. Mention has already been made of inactivation of gentamicin by carbenicillin and other penicillins[55][56] and the high incidence of nephrotoxicity with combinations of cephalothin

Table 3   Results of some studies of effects of combinations with rifampicin

Reference	Antibiotic used with rifampicin	Nature of study	Organisms	Observation recorded
78	(a) Fusidic acid	Effect on staphylococcal infections in man	Staph. aureus	(a) Rifampicin resistant strains emerged in 2/33 patients
	(b) Novobiocin			(b) Rifampicin resistant strains emerged in 1/6 patients
79	Erythromycin	(i) Treatment of a case of staphylococcal endocarditis	Staph. aureus	(i) Successful treatment
		(ii) *In vitro*: half chessboard titration		(ii) Bactericidal effect on the strain
80	Novobiocin	*In vitro*: chessboard titration on agar	Salm. typhi	Synergism with 17/18 strains
81	Tetracycline	Gram-negative infections in mice	S. typhimurium, E. coli, Pr. vulgaris, Sh. dysenteriae, Ps. aeruginosa	Synergism or addition
82	(a) Tetracycline (b) Benzyl penicillin (c) Streptomycin (d) Polymyxin B	(i) *In vitro* chessboard titration in liquid media (ii) Killing curves	Ps. aeruginosa (5) Pr. vulgaris (5) Pr. mirabilis (5)	(a) Combinations with tetracycline antagonistic with all 3 species (b) Combinations with benzyl penicillin or streptomycin antagonistic with Ps. aeruginosa indifferent with Proteus spp (c) Combination with polymyxin B synergistic with all 3 species

Table 3 (*cont.*)

				Addition
83	Polymyxin B	*In vitro* chessboard titration in liquid media	*Serratia marcescens* (12)	
23	Nalidixic Acid	(a) *In vitro* chessboard titration in liquid media (b) Turbidimetric studies (growth curves) (c) Bladder model	*E. coli* (2) *Pr. mirabilis* (2) *Ps. aeruginosa* (2) *Kl. aerogenes*	(a) **Little or no synergy with 8/8 strains** (b) and (c) Suppression of emergence of resistant mutants
87	Trimethoprim	*In vitro* chessboard titration on agar	(a) *Proteus* spp., *E. coli, Kl. aerogenes, Enterobacter* spp., *Ps. aeruginosa, B. fragilis, Salm. typhimurium, Streptococci* (280 strains) (b) *Staph. aureus* (24 strains)	(a) Synergism or addition in a high percentage (b) Antagonism in 24/24
88	Trimethoprim	*In vitro* chessboard titration on agar	*E. coli, Pr. mirabilis, Kl. aerogenes, Strept. faecalis, Staph. albus*	Synergism with 16/100 strains; no synergism with *Klebsiella* spp.
89	Trimethoprim	*In vitro* chessboard titration on agar	*Ps. aeruginosa, Citrobacter freundii, Proteus* spp., *Providencia* spp., *E. coli, Flavobacterium* spp. *E. cloacae, Acinetobacter* spp., *Klebsiella* spp.	No antagonism; synergism with 26/61 strains; useful synergism at serum levels with only 2 strains; useful synergism at urine level with 24/61 strains
24	Trimethoprim	*In vitro* steady state inhibition of growth rates	*Str. faecalis* (1) *Kl. aerogenes* (1)	Antagonism and suppression of emergence of rifampicin resistant mutants

and gentamicin[37]. The question of whether cephalosporins potentiate or antagonise aminoglycoside nephrotoxicity has been examined by Marsh[75 76]. The nephrotoxic side effects of the older aminoglycosides are well known and the results of trials in man generally support the suggestion that combinations of the aminoglycosides and cephalosporins, and in particular of gentamicin and cephalothin, are nephrotoxic. However, the results of animal experiments suggest that cephalosporins may prevent the development of the nephrotoxic effect which would otherwise result from aminoglycoside administration. However, as I have already pointed out, there are difficulties in using the animal model which may not always accurately reflect the effects in man. Therefore, at present it would seem wise to follow Marsh's recommendation to avoid prescribing an aminoglycoside and cephalosporin together wherever possible and, if the combination is used, to watch for the appearance of proteinuria and to monitor renal function.

Combinations of rifampicin and other antibacterial agents

Rifampicin has become a mainstay in the treatment of tuberculosis, but unlike isoniazid it is also active against Gram-positive and Gram-negative organisms. However, many people, fearing that its widespread use in the absence of other antituberculous drugs might result in the emergence of rifampicin resistant strains of *Mycobacterium tuberculosis*, believe that it should not be used for the treatment of non-mycobacterial illness.

In spite of these fears, the possibility of using rifampicin in combination with other antibacterial agents in the treatment of infections caused by Gram-positive and Gram-negative bacteria has been explored. Combination therapy is used in an effort to produce synergism and to reduce the risk of producing rifampicin resistant organisms which otherwise readily emerge. In 1977 I reviewed the literature and discussed the problem in general[77]. Table 3 shows some of the agents studied in combination with rifampicin and the effects that have been observed *in vitro* or in animals or man.

Fusidic acid and novobiocin each failed to prevent the emergence of rifampicin resistant staphylococci in clinical infections in man[78].

The combination of rifampicin and erythromycin was shown to be synergistic against a staphylococcus causing endocarditis and was successful in the treatment of the infection[79].

Novobiocin and rifampicin in concentrations readily obtainable in the bile were synergistic *in vitro* against 17 of 18 strains of *Salmonella typhi* and the suggestion has been made that because of rifampicin's intracellular activity this combination could be considered for the treatment of typhoid carriers[80].

Tetracycline and rifampicin were found to produce a synergistic or additive effect in Gram-negative infections in mice[81], but *in vitro* the same combination was found to be antagonistic against *Ps. aeruginosa, Proteus vulgaris* and *Proteus mirabilis*[82]. Rifampicin and benzyl penicillin or streptomycin were antagonistic with *Ps. aeruginosa,* but exhibited indifference with *Proteus* spp. Rifampicin and Polymyxin B were synergistic with all three species and additive with *Serratia marcescens*[83].

Little or no *in vitro* synergism could be demonstrated between nalidixic acid and rifampicin by chessboard titrations, but subinhibitory concentrations of each drug prevented the emergence of mutants resistant to the other and a combination of the two was suggested as a rational choice for the treatment of urinary infections[23].

The combination of rifampicin and trimethoprim has been extensively studied. All investigators apparently agree that the serum half-life of trimethoprim is significantly reduced by rifampicin, but they do not agree about the nature of other pharmacokinetic effects[84-86] nor is there agreement about the nature of the combined antibacterial effect. Using a chessboard technique on solid media several investigators found the combination to be synergistic against a wide variety of Gram-negative bacteria and streptococci and demonstrated antagonism only with *Staph. aureus*[87-89]. Although the methods were essentially the same the criteria for synergism varied to some extent as did the frequency with which it was observed. Nevertheless, in most cases explanations for discrepancies were apparent in that the sensitivity of the organisms under investigation to the individual components of the combination differed and some investigators deliberately selected high proportions of resistant organisms.

Unfortunately, a discordant note was sounded by Harvey[24]. Using one strain of *Strept. faecalis* and one of *Kl. aerogenes* with which synergism had been demonstrated by other investigators, but employing the measurement of steady state inhibition of specific growth rates by rifampicin alone and in combination as the indicator of the nature of the combined effect he designated it antagonism. In his view the experimental observations of the other investigators were correct, but their interpretation was not, the synergism they saw being apparent rather than real and due to the suppression by trimethoprim of mutants resistant to low concentrations of rifampicin. Furthermore, while other workers base their explanation for synergism upon the fact that rifampicin, by selectively inhibiting RNA polymerase and therefore transcription, can be regarded as acting upon the same metabolic pathway as trimethoprim, namely nucleic acid synthesis, and causing sequential blockade, Harvey regards the most likely effect of a combination of two such inhibitors as antagonism, and concludes that the suppression of rifampicin resistant mutants would be better achieved by tetracycline or erythromycin. Observers, be they experts or not, might feel justifiably confused by the disagreement. Unfortunately, they will gain little comfort from the fact that it is a clear demonstration of just how difficult it is to find a clear answer to a question about the nature of the effect of a combination of antibacterial agents.

CONCLUSIONS

When I was a newly qualified doctor I once had the temerity to ask a superior why he gave prophylactic penicillin routinely to all unconscious patients who had had a stroke since it appeared to do nothing to reduce the incidence of infection and indeed made the prognosis worse as the infections that did occur were with organisms resistant to penicillin and therefore more difficult to treat. I was told sharply that such patients were predisposed to infection and it was obvious that antibiotics were indicated. The episode taught me two lessons. First, what may be obvious may not be right, and second there are circumstances in which it is better to keep one's mouth shut. The second may have been the more valuable lesson, but the first is admirably demonstrated in the field of combined chemotherapy. It may seem 'obvious' that the administration of two active antimicrobial drugs will be twice as good as one, but each agent may adversely affect the properties of the other. Doubling the number of drugs may double or more than double the number and severity of side effects, and it is impossible to predict with certainty the effect of a combination upon a particular bacterial strain. If the condition of the patient is critical and if a combination is being considered it would seem wise to test its action against the infecting organism in the laboratory wherever possible, but unfortunately even this may not always provide a clear and unambiguous result.

It may be an overstatement to say that like beauty synergism is in the eye of the beholder, but different observers looking at the same combination may obtain different results or draw different conclusions, and the truth may not always be absolute.

References

1 Leading Article. (1978). Antibiotic antagonism and synergy. *Lancet*, **2,** 80
2 National Research Council Division of Medical Sciences Drug Efficacy Study (National Academy of Sciences). (1969). Fixed combinations of antimicrobial agents. *N. Engl. J. Med.*, **280,** 1149
3 Crout, J. R. (1974). Fixed combination prescription drugs: FDA policy. *J. Clin. Pharmacol.*, **14,** 249

4 Jawetz, E. and Gunnison, J. B. (1952). An experimental basis of combined antibiotic action. *J. Am. Med. Assoc.*, **150**, 693

5 Jawetz, E., Gunnison, J. B., Coleman, V. R. and Kempe, H. C. (1955). A laboratory test for bacterial sensitivity to combinations of antibiotics. *Am. J. Clin. Pathol.*, **25**, 1016

6 Bushby, S. R. M. and Hitchings, G. H. (1968). Trimethoprim, a sulphonamide potentiator. *Br. J. Pharmacol. Chemother.*, **33**, 72

7 Herman, L. G. (1959). Antibiotic sensitivity using pretreated plates. II. A demonstration of inhibitory activity with a low level combination of a sulphonamide and polymyxin B against *Proteus* species. *Antibiotics Annu.*, **1958–1959**, 836

8 Elek, S. D. and Hilson, G. R. F. (1954). Combined agar diffusion and replica plating techniques in the study of antibacterial substances. *J. Clin. Pathol.*, **7**, 37

9 Chabbert, Y. (1957). Une technique nouvelle d'étude de l'action bactéricide des associations d'antibiotiques: le transfer sur cellophane. *Ann. Inst. Pasteur*, **93**, 289

10 Garrod, L. P. and Waterworth, P. M. (1969). *Tests of Combined Antibacterial Action. ACP Broadsheet 63. May 1969*. (London: Association of Clinical Pathologists)

11 Dowling, H. F. (1957). Mixtures of antibiotics. *J. Am. Med. Assoc.*, **164**, 44

12 Weinstein, R. J., Young, L. S. and Hewitt, W. L. (1975). Comparison of methods for assessing *in vitro* antibiotic synergism against *Pseudomonas* and *Serratia J. Lab. Clin. Med.*, **86**, 853

13 Craig, W. A. and Kunin, C. M. (1973). Distribution of trimethoprim-sulphamethoxazole in tissues of Rhesus monkeys. *J. Infect Dis.*, **128** (Suppl.), 575

14 Böhni, E. (1969). Chemotherapeutic activity of the combination of trimethoprim and sulphamethoxazole in infections of mice. *Postgrad. Med. J. Suppl.* **45**, 18

15 Manten, A. and Meyerman-Wisse, M. J. (1961). Antagonism between antibacterial drugs. *Nature*, **192**, 671

16 Manten, A. and Meyerman-Wisse, M. J. (1962). A systematic study of antibiotic antagonism. *Antonie van Leeuwenhoek*, **28**, 321

17 Mouton, R. P. (1975). An introduction to aspects of synergism. In R. P. Mouton, W. Brumfitt and J. M. T. Hamilton-Miller (eds.) *The Rational Choice of Antibacterial Agents*, pp. 81–88. (London: Kluwer Harrap Handbooks)

18 Lacey, R. W. (1978). The suppression of the appearance of bacterial mutants by combined antibacterial therapy. *J. Antimicrob. Chemother.*, **4**, 391

19 Hamilton-Miller, J. M. T. and Brumfitt, W. (1975). Clinical aspects of *in vitro* antimicrobial synergism. In R. P. Mouton, W. Brumfitt and J. M. T. Hamilton-Miller (eds.) *The Rational Choice of Antibacterial Agents*, pp. 89–101. (London: Kluwer Harrap Handbooks)

20 Kaipainen, W. J. (1952). Effect of antibiotic combinations on bacterial resistance. *Ann. Med. Exp. Biol. Fenn.*, **30**, 61

21 Darrell, J. H., Garrod, L. P. and Waterworth, P. M. (1968). Trimethoprim: laboratory and clinical studies. *J. Clin. Pathol.*, **21**, 202

22 Emmerson, A. M. *et al.* (1978). Unpublished data cited by Reeves, D. S., Bint, A. J. and Bullock, D. W. Use of antibiotics. Sulphonamides, co-trimoxazole and tetracyclines. *Br. Med. J.*, **2**, 410

23 Greenwood, D. and Andrew, J. (1978). Rifampicin plus nalidixic acid: a rational combination for the treatment of urinary infection. *J. Antimicrob. Chemother.*, **4**, 533

24 Harvey, R. J. (1978). Antagonistic interaction of rifampicin and trimethoprim. *J. Antimicrob. Chemother.*, **4**, 315

25 Leigh, D. A., Simmons, K. and Norman, E. (1974). Bacterial flora of the appendix fossa in appendicitis and postoperative wound infection. *J. Clin. Pathol.*, **27**, 997
26 Ingham, H. R., Sisson, P. R., Tharagonnet, D., Selkon, J. B. and Codd, A. A. (1977). Inhibition of phagocytosis *in vitro* by obligate anaerobes. *Lancet*, **2**, 1252
27 Anderson, J. D. (1975). Factors that may prevent transfer of antibiotic resistance between Gram-negative bacteria in the gut. *J. Med. Microbiol.*, **8**, 83
26 Salem, A. R., Jackson, D. D. and McFadzean, J. A. (1975). An investigation of interactions between metronidazole ("Flagyl") and other antibacterial agents. *J. Antimicrob. Chemother.*, **1**, 387
29 Okubadejo, O. A. and Allen, J. (1975). Combined activity of clindamycin and gentamicin on *Bacteroides fragilis* and other bacteria. *J. Antimicrob. Chemother.*, **1**, 403
30 Fass, R. J., Rotilie, C. A. and Prior, R. B. (1974). Interaction of clindamycin and gentamicin *in vitro*. *Antimicrob. Agents Chemother.*, **7**, 582
31 Snyder, R. J., Wilkowske, C. J. and Washington, J. A. (1975). Bactericidal activity of combinations of gentamicin with penicillin or clindamycin against *Streptococcus mutans*. *Antimicrob. Agents Chemother.*, **8**, 333
32 Meers, P. D. (1973). Bacteroides infections. *Lancet*, **2**, 573
33 Storring, R. A., Jameson, B., McElwain, T. J., Wiltsaw, E., Spiers, A. S. D. and Gaya, H. (1977). Oral non-absorbed antibiotics prevent infection in acute non-lymphoblastic leukaemia. *Lancet*, **2**, 837
34 Watson, J. G. and Jameson, B. (1979). Antibiotic prophylaxis for patients in protective isolation. *Lancet*, **1**, 1183
35 Enno, A., Catowsky, D., Darrell, J., Goldman, J. M., Hows, J. and Galton, D. A. G. (1978). Co-trimoxazole for prevention of infection in acute leukaemia. *Lancet*, **2**, 395
36 Lowenthal, R. M., Grossman, L., Goldman, J. M., Storring, R. A., Buskard, N. A., Park, D. S., Spiers, A. S. D. and Galton, D. A. G. (1975). Granulocyte transfusions in treatment of infections in patients with acute leukaemia and aplastic anaemia. *Lancet*, **1**, 353
37 The European Organisation for Research on Treatment of Cancer International Antimicrobial Therapy Project Group. (1978). Three antibiotic regimens in the treatment of infection in febrile granulocytopenic patients with cancer. *J. Infect. Dis.*, **137**, 14
38 Tattersall, M. H. N., Spiers, A. S. D. and Darrell, J. H. (1972). Initial therapy with combination of five antibiotics in febrile patients with leukaemia and neutropenia. *Lancet*, **1**, 162
39 Falk, R. H., Gillett, A. P., Wise, R. and Melikian, V. (1977). Tobramycin and clindamycin in the treatment of febrile leukaemic patients. *J. Antimicrob. Chemother.*, **3**, 317
40 Papayannis, A. G., Thomopoulos, D., Voulgaris, E., Scliros, Ph. and Gardikas, C. (1977). Tobramycin-cephalothin treatment in leukaemic and neutropenic patients with severe infection. *J. Antimicrob. Chemother.*, **3**, 311
41 Jawetz, E., Gunnison, J. B., Speck, R. S. and Coleman, V. R. (1951). Studies on antibiotic synergism and antagonism. The interference of chloramphenicol with the action of penicillin. *Arch. Intern. Med.*, **87**, 349
42 Lepper, M. H. and Dowling, H. F. (1951). Treatment of pneumococcic meningitis with penicillin compared with penicillin plus aureomycin. *Arch. Intern. Med.*, **88**, 489
43 Wallace, J. F., Smith, R. H., Garcia, M. and Petersdorf, R. G. (1967). Studies on the pathogenesis of meningitis. VI. Antagonism between penicillin and

chloramphenicol in experimental pneumococcal meningitis. *J. Lab. Clin. Med.*, **70**, 408

44 Ahern, J. J. and Kirby, W. M. M. (1953). Lack of interference of aureomycin with penicillin in treatment of pneumococcic pneumonia. *Arch. Intern. Med.*, **91**, 197

45 Davis, W. M. (1954). Successful treatment of pneumococcal pneumonia with combination of chloramphenicol and penicillin. *Am. J. Med. Sci.*, **227**, 391

46 Donald, G. and McKendrick, W. (1968). The treatment of pyogenic meningitis. *J. Neurol. Neurosurg. Psychiat.*, **31**, 528

47 Forbes, J. A. (1962). Purulent meningitis: principles and results of revised standardised treatment in 281 cases. *Aust. Ann. Med.*, **11**, 92

48 Christie, A. B. (1974). The treatment of pyogenic bacterial meningitis. *Prescribers' J.*, **14**, 110

49 Lorber, J. (1974). Treatment of neonatal meningitis. *Prescribers' J.*, **16**, 82

50 Strasbaugh, L. J., Mandaleris, C. D., Sherertz, R. J. and Sande, M. A. (1975). *In vivo* antagonism between gentamicin and chloramphenicol in rabbits with Gram-negative meningitis. *Clin. Res.*, **23**, 312A

51 Rahal, J. J. (1978). Antibiotic combinations. The clinical relevance of synergy and antagonism. *Medicine*, **57**, 179

52 Seidl, L. G., Thornton, G. F., Smith, J. W. and Cluff, L. E. (1966). Studies on the epidemiology of adverse drug reactions. III. Reactions in patients on a general medical service. *Johns Hopkins Hosp. Bull.*, **119**, 229

53 Koch-Weser, J., Sidel, V. W., Federman, R. N., Kanarek, P., Finer, D. C. and Eaton, A. E. (1970). Adverse effects of sodium colistimethate. Manifestations and specific reaction rates during 317 courses of therapy. *Ann. Intern. Med.*, **72**, 857

54 Dowling, H. F. and Lepper, M. H. (1964). Hepatic reactions to tetracycline. *J. Am. Med. Assoc.*, **188**, 307

55 McLaughlin, J. E. and Reeves, D. S. (1971). Clinical and laboratory evidence for inactivation of gentamicin by carbenicillin. *Lancet*, **1**, 261

56 Noone, P. and Pattison, J. R. (1971). Therapeutic implications of interaction of gentamicin and penicillins. *Lancet*, **2**, 575

57 Lynn, B. (1974). Antibiotic incompatibilies and interactions. In J. Klastersky (ed.) *Clinical Use of Combinations of Antibiotics*, pp. 24–51. (London: Hodder and Stoughton)

58 Bushby, S. R. M. (1969). Combined antibacterial action *in vitro* of trimethoprim and sulphonamides. *Postgrad. Med. J.*, **45** (Suppl. Nov.), 10

59 Brumfitt, W. and Pursell, R. (1972). Double blind trial to compare ampicillin, cephalexin, co-trimoxazole and trimethoprim in treatment of urinary infection. *Br. Med. J.*, **2**, 673

60 Simmons, N. A. (1975). Antibiotic synergy. *J. Antimicrob. Chemother.*, **1**, 257

61 Sabath, L. D., Steinhauer, B. W. and Finland, M. (1963). Combined action of penicillin G with methicillin or oxacillin against *Staphylococcus aureus*. *N. Engl. J. Med.*, **268**, 284

62 Hamilton-Miller, J. M. T., Smith, J. T. and Knox, R. (1964). Potentiation of penicillin action by inhibition of penicillinase. *Nature*, **201**, 867

63 Sabath, L. D. and Abraham, E. P. (1964). Synergistic action of penicillins and cephalosporins against *Pseudomonas pyocyanea*. *Nature*, **204**, 1066

64 Sutherland, R. and Batchelor, F. R. (1964). Synergistic activity of penicillins against penicillinase-producing Gram-negative bacilli. *Nature*, **201**, 868

65 Garau, J. and Kabins, S. A. (1979). Enhanced activity of ampicillin by oxacillin against enterococci. *J. Antimicrob. Chemother.*, **5**, 31

66 Neu, H. C. (1976). Synergy of Mecillinam, a beta-amidinopenicillanic acid

derivative, combined with beta-lactam antibiotics. *Antimicrob. Agents Chemother.*, **10**, 535

67 Grunberg, E., Cleland, R., Beskid, G. and DeLorenzo, W. F. (1976). *In vivo* synergy between 6 β-amidinopenicillanic acid derivatives and other antibiotics. *Antimicrob. Agents Chemother.*, **9**, 589

68 Pines, A., Nandi, A. R., Raafat, H. and Rahman, M. (1977). Pivmecillinam and amoxycillin as combined treatment in purulent exacerbations of chronic bronchitis. *J. Antimicrob. Chemother.*, **3** (Suppl. B), 141

69 Shanson, D. C., Brigden, W. and Weaver, E. J. M. (1977). *Salmonella enteritidis* endocarditis. *Br. Med. J.*, **1**, 612

70 Watt, B. (1978). Streptococcal endocarditis: a penicillin alone or a penicillin with an aminoglycoside? *J. Antimicrob. Chemother.*, **4**, 107

71 Jawetz, E. and Gunnison, J. B. (1950). The determination of sensitivity to penicillin and streptomycin of enterococci and streptococci of the viridans group. *J. Lab. Clin. Med.*, **35**, 488

72 Garrod, L. P. (1953). Combined chemotherapy in bacterial infections. *Br. Med. J.*, **1**, 953

73 Farrell, W., Wilks, M. and Drasar, F. A. (1979). Synergy between aminoglycosides and semi-synthetic penicillins against Gentamicin-resistant Gram-negative rods. *J. Antimicrob. Chemother.*, **5**, 23

74 Bulger, R. J. and Kirby, W. M. M. (1963). Gentamicin and ampicillin. Synergism with other antibiotics. *Am. J. Med. Sci.*, **246**, 717

75 Marsh, F. P. (1978). Do cephalosporins potentiate or antagonise aminoglycoside nephrotoxicity? *J. Antimicrob. Chemother.*, **4**, 103

76 Marsh, F. P. (1978). Do cephalosporins potentiate or antagonise aminoglycoside nephrotoxicity? *J. Antimicrob. Chemother.*, **4**, 577

77 Simmons, N. A. (1977). Synergy and rifampicin. *J. Antimicrob. Chemother.*, **3**, 109

78 Jensen, K. (1968). Methicillin resistant staphylococci. *Lancet*, **2**, 1078

79 Peard, M. C., Fleck, D. G., Garrod, L. P. and Waterworth, P. M. (1970). Combined rifampicin and erythromycin for bacterial endocarditis. *Br. Med. J.*, **4**, 410

80 Shanson, D. C. and Leung, T. (1976). Susceptibility of *Salmonella typhi* to rifamycins and novobiocin. *J. Antimicrob. Chemother.*, **2**, 81

81 Arioli, V., Pallanza, R., Nicolis, F. B. and Furesz, S. (1970). Experimental data on the interaction between rifampicin and tetracycline. *Progress in Antimicrobial and Anticancer Chemotherapy. Proceedings of the 6th International Congress of Chemotherapy*, p. 339. (Tokyo: University of Tokyo Press)

82 Perez Urena, M. T., Barasoain, I., Espinoza, M., Garcia, E. and Portoles, A. (1975). Evaluation of different antibiotic actions combined with rifampicin. *Chemotherapy*, **21**, 82

83 Traub, W. H. and Kleber, I. (1975). *In vitro* additive effect of polymyxin B and rifampicin against *Serratia marcescens*. *Antimicrob. Agents Chemother.*, **7**, 874

84 Hamilton-Miller, J. M. T. and Brumfitt, W. (1976). Trimethoprim and rifampicin: pharmacokinetic studies in man. *J. Antimicrob. Chemother.*, **2**, 181

85 Acocella, G. and Scotti, R. (1976). Kinetic studies on the combination rifampicin-trimethoprim in man. Absorption and urinary excretion after administration to healthy volunteers of single doses of the two compounds alone and in combination, and the combination over a period of one week. *J. Antimicrob. Chemother.*, **2**, 271

86 Emmerson, A. M., Grüneberg, R. N. and Johnson, E. S. (1978). The pharmacokinetics in man of a combination of rifampicin and trimethoprim. *J. Antimicrob. Chemother.*, **4**, 523

87 Kerry, D. W., Hamilton-Miller, J. M. T. and Brumfitt, W. (1975). Trimethoprim and rifampicin: *in vitro* activities separately and in combination. *J. Antimicrob. Chemother.*, **1**, 417
88 Grüneberg, R. N. and Emmerson, A. M. (1977). The interactions between rifampicin and trimethoprim: an *in vitro* study. *J. Antimicrob. Chemother.*, **3**, 453
89 Farrell, W., Wilks, M. and Drasar, F. A. (1977). The action of trimethoprim and rifampicin in combination against Gram-negative rods resistant to gentamicin. *J. Antimicrob. Chemother.*, **3**, 459
90 Brumfitt, W., Percival, A. and Leigh, D. A. (1967). Clinical and laboratory studies with carbenicillin. *Lancet*, **1**, 1289
91 Lin, M. Y. C., Tuazon, C. U. and Sheagren, J. N. (1979). Synergism of aminoglycosides and carbenicillin against resistant strains of *Serratia marcescens*. *J. Antimicrob. Chemother.*, **5**, 37
92 Watanakunakorn, C. and Glotzbecker, C. (1979). *In vitro* activity of carbenicillin, ticarcillin, aminoglycosides and combinations against *Staphylococcus aureus*. *J. Antimicrob. Chemother.*, **5**, 151

7

Antibiotic policies

J. B. Selkon

The increasing number of antibiotics, and a growing awareness of the problems arising from their use, have stimulated many attempts to develop policies to control and improve their usage. Despite numerous attempts, there has been a notable lack of success in developing a policy which has been widely accepted. The main reason for this has been the conflict between the medical ethic that the individual patient should receive the treatment most appropriate to his particular needs and the limitation of prescribing freedom imposed by policies, the main objective of which has been to protect the community as a whole from the emergence of drug-resistant bacteria. A secondary reason for this failure has been the excessive regimentation of prescribing imposed by policies which had, as their main objective, the application of rules to what was assumed to be *laissez-faire* chaos and thus inherently bad prescribing practice. Clinical experience has, however, frequently demonstrated the limitation of such policies and, as a result, they rapidly lost credibility. It is important, therefore, in developing an antibiotic policy to consider in detail the reasons for such a policy and to design it to achieve only specific and attainable objectives. This must be done with due consideration for the particular needs of the individual patient. Now that considerably more antibacterial agents are available, and there is an adequate choice, it may be possible to suggest, at least, the basic structure of such an antibiotic policy. However, first it is necessary to consider in detail the objectives and the limitations of antibiotic policies.

SIMPLIFICATION OF PATIENT MANAGEMENT

There are a number of admirable reviews of antimicrobial agents and

193

chemotherapy, from the comprehensive[1] to the brief[2]. Nevertheless, the multiplicity of available antibiotics now presents the clinician with the need either to digest a large body of information which is additional to his primary speciality, or to restrict his choice of antibacterial chemotherapy to only a limited number of agents.

An example of the latter is the simple prescribing chart described by Geddes[3]. Without considering specific criticisms of the individual antibiotics recommended by this author, there is the general criticism of this and other such policies, that they may be oversimplistic and as such fail to provide the most effective chemotherapy which would otherwise be available if the individual needs of the patients were fully considered. This is particularly important when considering seriously ill patients, where the initial chemotherapy must be effective against all the likely pathogenic organisms often before the results of laboratory tests are available. For example, if such a prescribing chart were used, a patient presenting with fulminating pneumonia, which could be due to *Staphylococcus aureus* or *Klebsiella* spp., would not receive flucloxacillin plus an aminoglycoside, or cefuroxime, the two alternative regimens which would otherwise have been considered the most appropriate treatment in this situation. Thus, by generalising, an antibiotic policy, though suitable for the majority, would provide an individual patient with suboptimal chemotherapy.

It is possible to produce more detailed recommendations than the example presented, but in order to do so they would have to be integrated into an overall policy designed to include the medical and surgical aspects of the management of the patient, and the microbiological diagnostic procedures to be undertaken. It is important to appreciate that the choice of chemotherapeutic agent is, to a large extent, dependent on patient factors. Thus, the site and extent of the lesion, the presence of pus, renal and hepatic function and the immunological state of the patient must all be considered. Such a policy must also specify at which point specialist advice on antimicrobial chemotherapy should be sought. This, far from being a simple guide to antimicrobial chemotherapy, then becomes a complex operational procedure, which is only applicable to a unit or subunit of a particular speciality and depends on the continued interest and cooperation of the physicians, surgeons and microbiologists concerned. Furthermore, it is essential that the use of such operational policies are associated with the active education of all new junior medical staff and that they are subject to regular review. This involves detailed consultation between clinicians and microbiologists concerning the clinical effectiveness of any recommendations, changes in procedure in the unit or laboratory, and the emergence of drug resistant organisms. Although policies orientated to the clinical needs of a particular speciality should give the patient the advantage of the most appropriate and effective antimicrobial chemotherapy, the implementation of such policies are so time-consuming as to be impractical except by a limited number of specialised departments. They are definitely not a means of simplifying medical practice and, in conclusion, it is suggested that this is not an attainable objective of an antibiotic policy.

CONTROL AND PREVENTION OF THE EMERGENCE OF DRUG-RESISTANT BACTERIA

The second objective of an antibiotic policy is to protect the community from the emergence and spread of drug-resistant bacteria[4] [5]. This is particularly relevant in hospital practice where nosocomial infections are said to account for up to 10% of hospital care[6]. The spread of drug resistant organisms in such a community can diminish the effectiveness of previously useful antibiotics and lead to an increase in morbidity and mortality in susceptible patients. Drug resistance may arise by various mechanisms, for example mutation, which may be a slow process involving a sequence of 'small step' mutations with a gradual increase in resistance, or, as is the case of resistance to the aminoglycosides, erythromycin and fusidic acid, by a single-step mutation, leading to the growth of highly resistant organisms. Policies have been suggested which either restrict the use of such antibiotics[7], or use them only as part of a double-drug regime[8]-[10]. The former proposal could be questioned on ethical grounds, since it may deprive the individual patient of the most effective treatment. A more acceptable policy is to restrict the use of such agents to a hospital isolation unit equipped to prevent nosocomial infection. An area in which a policy of absolute restriction is justifiable is in the use of topical antibiotics, which should be strictly limited, in hospital practice, to those agents which are never used systemically. The double- or triple-drug regime has been used for many years in the treatment of tuberculosis, where it has been shown that the small numbers of naturally occurring mutants are favourably selected by a single-drug treatment. Although with non-tuberculous infection there still remains reasonable doubt of the effectiveness of a double-drug regime, and, in some instances this type of regime may only delay the emergence of resistance[11], it has sufficient support[12] to be an acceptable recommendation.

Drug resistant bacteria may also emerge as the result of the spread of plasmid-borne genes. An example is penicillin resistance in staphylococci, which is due not to mutation but to the acquisition of a plasmid-borne gene conveying the ability to synthesise β-lactamase and the selection of such strains by the antibiotic environment of the hospital. This is the main method for the spread of drug resistance in Gram-negative bacilli which are the main cause of hospital acquired infection today. The drug resistant plasmids not only divide and multiply with the bacterial cell, but under favourable circumstances can be transferred to other bacteria of the same or related species, by conjugation or transduction. In this way, resistance to antibiotics may be transferred from commensal organisms to those causing serious infections. These resistant organisms multiply in an environment in which there is a widespread use of antibiotics, particularly those with a broad spectrum of activity. In the absence of antibiotics, they appear to be at a slight metabolic disadvantage compared with non-plasmid-bearing organisms and the number of antibiotic-sensitive organisms gradually increases. Therefore, one of the most important aspects of antibiotic policy should be to eliminate, as far as possible, the non-essential use of antibiotics. Sheckler and Bennett[13] showed that 62% of patients receiving antibiotics had no evidence of infection, and Kayser[14], in a study of a 500 bed hospital in Switzerland, provided evidence which suggests that 39% of patients in hospital were prescribed antibiotics unnecessarily. This was mainly attributed to chemoprophylaxis for surgery, despite the limited number of conditions in which it has been proved to be beneficial. It is important to realise that these include only the prevention of endocarditis in patients with rheumatic or congenital heart disease following dental surgery or tonsillectomy; clostridial infection in patients with peripheral vascular disease; and infection following surgery of the large bowel, open-heart and brain surgery. However, in most other instances it is of doubtful value and may even do more harm than good[15].

The beneficial effect of the withdrawal of antibiotics on the prevalence of drug-resistant bacteria in a unit or hospital has been demonstrated repeatedly. Thus, Barber *et al.*[12] showed that in one specific hospital, the prevalence of penicillin-resistant staphylococci progressively fell when penicillin was withdrawn from routine usage. Price and Sleigh[16] reported on the disappearance of multiply drug resistant strains of *Klebsiella aerogenes* from a neurosurgical unit after the withdrawal of all antibiotics. Thus, the removal of the ecological pressure in favour of drug-resistant strains is a reasonable objective of an antibiotic policy. It has been suggested that this can be achieved by rotation of antibiotic usage, though in practice this is difficult to implement. It is theoretically simpler to recommend instead that the use of the broad spectrum antibiotics such as the cephalosporins be radically restricted and that the ecological pressures in favour of the selection of specific resistant organisms be reduced by the use of different groups of antibiotics. For example, the restriction of the use of co-trimoxazole to infections of the urinary tract, and the restriction of ampicillin to infections of the respiratory tract and appropriate wound infections would be less likely to select a resistant flora than the use of either of these agents for both urinary, respiratory and wound infections. Thus, diversity of chemotherapeutic agents should be considered as one of the principles of an antibiotic policy. Evidence of the danger of limiting the range of antibiotics available to clinicians is afforded by the experience in Czechoslovakia[17] where a national antibiotic policy of a very limited number of antibiotics has been associated with much higher prevalences of drug resistance than are seen in hospitals in the United Kingdom.

ADVERSE REACTIONS TO ANTIBIOTICS

The serious adverse effects of antibiotics have been well documented. Thus, one 3 year study[18] found the risk of these reactions to range from 0.88% to 8.5% for various antimicrobial agents, with an overall risk of 4.5%. The majority of drug reactions were not mild or trivial, 58% being moderate to severe, either requiring therapy, extending hospital stay, or threatening the patient's life. This provides substantial additional support for restraint in prescribing antimicrobial agents.

COST OF CHEMOTHERAPY

Economy in the medical services is always a desirable objective and the cost of antibacterial chemotherapy forms an appreciable part of hospital budgets. Studies in the USA[19] [23] have shown that approximately one third or more of a hospital's pharmaceutical budget is expended on antibiotics. Roberts and Visconti[24] found that 77% of their hospital's antimicrobial expenditure was for irrational chemotherapy and, of this, 80% was for chemophrophylaxis on surgical wards; the irrational chemotherapy was responsible for 92% of all adverse drug effects.

A great deal of argument is often generated over the relative costs of different antimicrobial agents. There are a few examples where much cheaper agents would be as effective as very expensive antibiotics. For example, flucloxacillin at £0.50 per day would, in nearly all instances, be as effective as fusidic acid at £3.00 per day. Similarly, gentamicin at £5.00 per day has a clear-cut advantage over amikacin at £38.00 per day, except when treating gentamicin-resistant but amikacin-sensitive strains of *Pseudomonas*. There is also neither therapeutic nor financial merit in using cefoxitin (£36.00 per day) instead of the combination of intravenous metronidazole plus either ampicillin (£11.00) or gentamicin at £15.00 per day. With regard to the smaller differences of costs of many other agents and particularly for patients in hospital, where the saving of one day's bed usage far outweighs the cost of antimicrobial agents, there is little to be gained provided the chemotherapy was definitely required for treatment. In the absence of true cost accounting, which takes into account the duration of bed stay and the relative effectiveness of agents, it is economically advisable to choose the most effective bactericidal agent with the exception of the most expensive agents referred to above.

In summary, it would seem that the prime consideration with respect to the costs of chemotherapeutic agents should be the reduction of unnecessary chemotherapy. There is an advantage to be gained from limiting the use of the very expensive agents, namely fusidic acid, amikacin, cefoxtin and the cephalosporins, but this would be of considerably smaller benefit.

CONCLUSION

The above arguments suggest that an antibiotic policy which is merely a simple guide to antibacterial chemotherapy will be of little value and that complex guides to treatment, though applicable locally to specialities, would not be widely acceptable. The main objective of an antibiotic policy is, therefore, to prevent and control the emergence of drug resistant bacteria, and this must be done without preventing the individual patient from receiving the highest standard of treatment. It is suggested that this may be achieved by adhering to the following principles:

(1) *Education* – The essential requirement of an antibiotic policy is continuing education, both through formal lectures and through daily advice and discussion of individual patients.

(2) *Restriction* – As stated by Williams *et al.*[25], the first principle governing the use of antibiotics within a hospital should be the rigid restriction to really necessary indications, in order that a resistant bacterial population may not be bred and disseminated. This dictum should be extended to restrict the use of antibiotics to which resistance rapidly emerges, namely fusidic acid, the aminoglycosides and erythromycin.

(3) *Combined chemotherapy* – This should be recommended when fusidic acid, the aminoglycosides or erythromycin have to be used in hospital.

(4) *Diversification of chemotherapy* – Diversification of the antimicrobial environment of the hospital is a desirable objective and is most easily achieved by restricting co-trimoxazole for the treatment of infections of the urinary tract only and ampicillin for infections of the lower respiratory tract. The broad spectrum antibiotics, cephalosporins and cephamycins should not be used for chemoprophylaxis.

(5) *Surveillance* – An antibiotic policy must be associated with continual bacteriological surveillance for the emergence of drug resistant strains and their detection followed by effective isolation and containment.

DEVELOPMENT AND MANAGEMENT OF ANTIBIOTIC POLICIES

The methods of development of antibiotic policies and their management in the USA have been thoroughly reviewed and discussed[26]. In the USA, all hospitals accredited to the Joint Commission on the Accreditation of Hospitals have had to institute medical staff reviews of antibiotic usage. Alternatively, they have established multidisciplinary committees composed of representatives of the clinical departments, pharmacy and hospital administration to consider antibiotic utilization. However, there is no evidence that these approaches have been effective in reducing unnecessary or inappropriate chemotherapy and, in view of the diversity of opinion among doctors, it would be surprising if such committees could in many ways be effective. They certainly would be so time consuming of medical man-hours as to be counter-productive and unacceptable to the medical profession in the United Kingdom.

Other procedures which have been used in the USA are those that have required either special consultation or written justification before antibiotics on a restricted list can be prescribed[22]. The omission of agents from the hospital pharmacy's formulary has also been suggested but this would only be acceptable in the United Kingdom for similar antibiotics in which equivalence has been proven.

In the Newcastle General Hospital a simple antibiotic policy has been carried out for over a decade. Clinicians reserve the right to prescribe whatever antibiotic they think appropriate. When antibiotics are prescribed which are on the list prepared by the Control of Infection Officer (C.I.O.) as potentially liable to give rise to the emergence of drug resistant bacteria, this information is conveyed by internal post to the C.I.O. by the pharmacist using a simple form. At present, the list consists of fusidic acid, erythromycin, clindamycin, gentamicin, tobramycin, amikacin and all cephalosporins. Within a few days the

C.I.O. discusses with the clinician concerned the control of infection aspects of the antibiotic that he has prescribed and he is left to continue or discontinue its use as he thinks appropriate. Thus, the clinician has complete freedom of action. This policy has worked effectively and the joint consultations have been valuable to both parties in updating the knowledge necessary for rational prescribing and the awareness of the real clinical problems that are encountered. An assessment of the effectiveness of this approach, though imprecise, is afforded by the number of doses of the following antibiotics which were prescribed during 1978 in this 1000 bed acute district general hospital containing a major accident department, a regional burns unit and an intensive care unit: gentamicin 3200×0.08 g and 1200×0.02 g, amikacin 195×0.5 g, tobramycin – nil, cefoxitin – nil, cefuroxime 360×0.75 g, fusidic acid 110×0.5 g i.v., and 5500×0.25 g orally. Alternatively, these amounts may be expressed as a proportion of the 26 000 patients admitted during 1978.

It is suggested that the only antibiotic policy which would and should be accepted is a local one which would embrace no more than a hospital district or equivalent administrative unit. Secondly, that such a policy should be developed and implemented, possibly by a committee, but preferably by a doctor who is also responsible for the control of hospital acquired infections. Time which is so frequently wasted in committee may be better employed in consultation on specific clinical problems since it is from these discussions that a realistic antibiotic policy can be developed and the necessary mutual education take place.

References

1 Garrod, L. P., Lambert, H. P. and O'Grady, F. (1973). *Antibiotics and Chemotherapy*. (Edinburgh: Churchill Livingstone)
2 Regional Microbiology Subcommittee. (1979). *A Guide to the Use of Antimicrobial Drugs*. (South East Thames Regional Health Authority)
3 Geddes, A. M. (1977). *Prescribers' Journal*. 17, 124
4 Jackson, G. G. (1979). Antibiotic policies, practices and pressures (Leading article). *J. Antimicrob. Chemother.*, 5, 1
5 Buckwold, F. J. and Ronald, R. (1979). Antimicrobial misuse – effects and suggestions for control. *J. Antimicrob. Chemother.*, 5, 129
6 Freeman, J. (1977). *J. Clin. Res.*, 25, 264
7 Lowbury, E. J. L., Ayliffe, G. A. J., Geddes, A. M. and Williams, J. D. (1975). *Control of Hospital Infection*, p. 191. (London: Chapman and Hall)
8 Barber, M. (1963). Antibiotics and hospital infection. In Williams, R. E. O. and Shooter, R. A. (eds.) *Infection in Hospitals*, p. 289. (Oxford: Blackwell)
9 Jensen, K. and Lassen, H. C. A. (1969). Combined treatment with antibacterial chemotherapeutical agents in staphylococcal infections. *Q. J. Med.*, 38, 91

10 Brumfitt, W. and Percival, A. (1971). Antibiotic Combinations (Occasional Survey). *Lancet*, **1**, 387

11 Lowbury, E. J. L. (1957). Chemotherapy for *Staphylococcus aureus*. Combined use of novobiocin and erythromycin and other methods in the treatment of burns. *Lancet*, **2**, 305

12 Barber, M., Dutton, A. A. C., Beard, M. A., Elmes, P. C. and Williams, R. (1960). Reversal of antibiotic resistance in hospital staphylococcal infections. *Br. Med. J.*, **1**, 11

13 Scheckler, W. E. and Bennett, J. V. (1970). Antibiotic usage in seven community hospitals. *J. Am. Med. Assoc.*, **213**, 264

14 Kayser, F. H. (1978). Use of antimicrobial drugs in general hospitals and in general practice. In *Current Chemotherapy: Proceedings 10th Int. Congress Chemotherapy*, Zurich, 1977. *Am. Soc. Microbiol.*, **2**, 36

15 Taylor, G. W. (1960). Preventive use of antibiotics in surgery. *Br. Med. Bull.*, **16**, 51

16 Price, D. J. E. and Sleigh, J. D. (1970). Control of infection due to *Klebsiella aerogenes* in a neurosurgical unit by withdrawal of all antibiotics. *Lancet*, **2**, 1213

17 Modr, Z. (1978). Antibiotic policy in Czechoslovakia. *J. Antimicrob. Chemother.*, **4**, 305

18 Caldwell, J. R. and Cluff, L. E. (1974). Adverse reactions to antimicrobial agents. *J. Am. Med. Assoc.*, **230**, 77

19 Kunin, C. M., Tupasi, T. and Craig, W. A. (1973). Use of antibiotics. A brief exposition of the problem and some tentative solutions. *Ann. Intern. Med.*, **79**, 555

20 Simmons, H. E. and Stolley, P. D. (1974). This is medical progress? Trends and consequences of antibiotic use in the United States. *J. Am. Med. Assoc.*, **227**, 1023

21 Zeman, B. T., Pike, M. and Samet, C. (1974). The antibiotic utilization committee. *Hospitals*, **48**, 73

22 McGowan, J. E. and Finland, M. (1974). Infection and antibiotic usage at Boston City Hospital: changes in prevalence during the decade 1964–73. *J. Infect. Dis.*, **129**, 421

23 Kunin, C. M. (1978). Use of antimicrobial drugs in general hospitals and in general practice. In *Current Chemotherapy: Proceedings 10th Int. Congress Chemotherapy*, Zurich, 1977. *Am. Soc. Microbiol.*, **2**, 36

24 Roberts, A. W. and Visconti, J. A. (1972). The rational and irrational use of systemic antimicrobial drugs. *Am. J. Hosp. Pharm.*, **29**, 828

25 Williams, R. E. O., Blowers, R., Garrod, L. P. and Shooter, R. A. (1966). *Hospital Infection, Causes and Prevention*, p. 213. (London: Lloyd-Luke)

26 Counts, G. W. (1977). Review and control of antimicrobial usage in hospitalized patients: A recommended collaborative approach (Special Communication). *J. Am. Med. Assoc.*, **238**, 2170

8

Antibiotic prescribing policies: a personal view

R. N. Grüneberg

There is no field of medical treatment which more directly invites intervention from outside than does antimicrobial chemotherapy. This is so for a number of reasons: firstly, because the choice of drugs is so bewilderingly large that clinicians, who have to be experts in many other areas, rarely use antibiotics to the best clinical advantage; secondly, because antimicrobial therapy leads to an accumulation of resistant bacteria; thirdly, because antibiotics are expensive; and fourthly, because there is available another group of specialists, the medical microbiologists, some of whom have the interest and knowledge to try and help their clinical colleagues. The first three of these reasons give an indication of the possible objectives of antibiotic policies, the fourth shows a possible avenue by which they can be introduced, modified and monitored.

OBJECTIVES OF ANTIBIOTIC POLICIES

(i) Appropriate choice of antibiotic for the individual patient
The wellbeing of the patient should always be the over-riding aim of treatment. The difficulty is to make an appropriate choice among the many possibilities. Clinicians generally are badly informed about antimicrobial drugs and receive a great deal of confusing and biased 'guidance' from the pharmaceutical industry; it is difficult enough for the interested 'expert' to assess the claims made for the many new products as they are introduced, and almost impossible for busy clinicians. Clearly, there is a need for the experts to guide their colleagues. This can be done in general terms by sending out a stream of

circulars, or more specifically by seeing the patients and offering guidance. The advice given will be concerned with choice of drugs, dosage, route and frequency of administration, drug interactions, possible side effects and many other such considerations. This latter approach is only defensible if the expert sees the patient, reviews the circumstances of the infection concerned and commits himself to a view which is recorded in the patient's notes. If the clinician then takes the proffered advice he does so knowing that the responsibility has been shared.

Two main kinds of problem are encountered: undertreatment and overtreatment. Undertreatment is not very common, but is most usually exemplified, in my experience, by the cautious attitude of many doctors to the aminoglycoside group of drugs. Drugs such as gentamicin are potential lifesavers, and should be used as such. Often, the clinician is so concerned about the possibility of toxicity that enough gentamicin is not given. The function of the expert is to make sure that the dosage is adequate to treat the life-threatening infection and to make sure that the blood levels are monitored. He should also give guidance about that most difficult clinical decision, when to stop treatment. His advice will be to treat serious infections seriously, and to be prepared to accept a price in possible unwanted side effects in return for survival of the patient. It is depressing in the extreme to read case reports[1] of patients dying from undertreated sepsis because of the anxiety of clinicians to avoid risking the development of infrequent side effects. Sometimes valuable drugs are virtually completely discarded for this inappropriate reason – chloramphenicol being a good example. The job of the expert should be to help the clinician by restoring a sense of proportion to the consideration of risks and benefits.

Overtreatment is much commoner. Either a sledgehammer is being used to crack a nut, or an antibiotic is being used when none is needed. Good prescribing in antimicrobial therapy, as in any other drug treatment, should embody the principle of economy of effort. No more treatment should be given than is strictly necessary. Far and away the biggest problem here is the use of antibiotics when none are needed. This ranges from the widespread abuse of antimicrobial prophylaxis (reviewed in Chapter 2), to the energetic treatment of trivial and self-limiting infection. The first rule of clinical care is to cause no harm to the patient. Any decision about the use of antibiotics must, therefore, weigh the possible benefits against the possible harm. If the possible benefit is slight, treatment should be adjusted accordingly. The possible harm may accrue to the patient in the form of unwanted side effects, to the community at large in the accumulation of unwanted antibiotic resistance or to both in the form of unwanted expenditure. The most frequent piece of advice on chemotherapy which I give to my clinical colleagues when I see their patients is to stop all antibiotics.

When it is clear that the patient is infected but not yet clear what the pathogen is, or what its sensitivities to antibiotics may be, it may be necessary to make decisions on antimicrobial choice on a 'best guess' basis. This requires up to date information on the drug sensitivities of relevant pathogens in the neighbourhood. This is important because drug sensitivities vary from place to place and from time to time. Illustrative observations on the sensitivities of urinary pathogens isolated in my own laboratory are presented in Table 1. It can be seen, for instance, that the usefulness of co-trimoxazole, nalidixic acid, sulphonamides and tetracyclines in hospital has been well maintained, but that there has been a progressive decline in the effectiveness of ampicillin/amoxycillin and of the cephalosporins. Familiarity with such information locally greatly strengthens the position of a clinical microbiologist offering drug advice. The microbiologist will also know something of the prevalence of infections with various organisms locally, and will be in a position to give due weight (and no more) to reports emanating from his own laboratory.

(ii) Choice of antibiotic to minimise the development of resistance

Drug resistance is a major consideration in antibiotic policy. Various approaches have been used, but much the most important is simply to reduce the amount or number of antibiotic(s) prescribed. As indicated above by Dr Selkon, the effect of antibiotic restriction may not only be to reduce the resistance of pathogens but also to reduce the prevalence of infection. Other tactics employed (reviewed in Chapter 7) include the combination of drugs in the hope of delaying the emergence of resistance, reduction of drug dosage or the time for which the drug is taken, rotation of antibiotics or the use of a large number of different agents. All of these ploys have their adherents. The basis of all of these approaches is scientifically somewhat shaky but these tactics are all that we have to guide us at present.

When the situation gets out of hand and resistant organisms become prevalent, logically devised antibiotic restriction policies may correct the difficulty[2 3]. Such solutions to emergent problems are not as satisfactory as preventing outbreaks of resistance from occurring. Big contributions to prevention of resistance could be made by stopping the use of chemotherapy which is not indicated, notably in unwarranted antimicrobial prophylaxis and in the use of topical chemotherapy.

It is not sufficiently realised that it is only rarely that the organism causing the infection becomes resistant during chemotherapy. Much more usually, it is harmless commensal organisms which are exposed incidentally during chemotherapy which become antibiotic resistant. These organisms subsequently become part of the flora from which new infecting strains will be derived; for example, some antimicrobials when given by mouth are more likely than others to generate resistance in the bowel flora[4], the source of urinary pathogens. This may happen either because the faecal organisms develop resistance or because the original sensitive organisms are replaced by more resistant strains or species. An example is the replacement of antibiotic-sensitive coliforms by the more antibiotic resistant *Klebsiella* spp. or *Pseudomonas aeruginosa* as a result of ampicillin/amoxycillin or cephalosporin use. Since such replacement is particularly undesirable in areas such as Intensive Care Units or Premature Baby Units, a 'house rule' has been instituted at University College Hospital banning the use of these drugs in such areas. As has been pointed out[5] such rules, or indeed antibiotic policies as a whole, can only have local relevance and must be kept under continuing review in the light of changing circumstances.

Table 1   Sensitivity of all urinary pathogens to various drugs 1971–78

Drug	*Percentage of strains fully sensitive in the years:*				
	1971	1973	1975	1977	1978
(A) General practice					
Amoxycillin	88.2	82.4	83.7	80.9	79.4
Cephalexin	87.5	86.6	84.4	82.9	84.5
Co-trimoxazole	96.6	94.9	95.0	95.7	97.0
Nalidixic acid	90.7	88.2	85.9	83.8	85.5
Sulphonamide	76.4	75.6	76.9	74.1	73.6
Tetracycline	72.5	73.3	74.7	75.0	75.7
(B) Hospital practice					
Amoxycillin	66.1	66.6	63.2	63.2	51.2
Cephalexin	69.9	68.7	69.3	64.3	58.2
Co-trimoxazole	83.9	82.2	81.3	86.3	82.5
Nalidixic acid	84.8	81.6	82.5	77.1	85.5
Sulphonamide	61.9	67.7	64.4	63.5	58.5
Tetracycline	55.8	53.4	54.2	56.8	59.3

(iii) Choice of antibiotic according to cost

It must be re-iterated that the first requirement of chemotherapy is to select the most appropriate treatment for the individual patient. Nonetheless, economy of expenditure is a desirable aim, whether the patient, an insurance company or the taxpayer are paying the bill. When other considerations are equal, the cheapest antibiotic should be preferred. As it happens, it is often true that the most clinically appropriate drug is also the cheapest, so that objective (i) (above) and objective (iii) are well matched.

It is not possible to give costs for drugs which are correct for long, or which are appropriate for both general practice and hospital use, or which are transferable from one hospital to another, or which apply in all countries. Accordingly the observations which I now make are made in the light of prices ruling at University College Hospital as I write.

For urinary tract infection, in general practice, almost any of the usually used 'urinary' antibiotics will give a similar cure rate, about 85–90%. There is little to choose between them on efficacy, so cost is a legitimate factor in choice. The cost of a 5 day course in standard dosage of some of the usual drugs is shown in Table 2.

In hospital urinary tract infection why use co-trimoxazole (£1.26 for 5 days) if the organism is sulphonamide sensitive, when a sulphonamide costs only 12p?

Incidentally, if the nitrofurantoin had been prescribed not by its

Table 2 Cost of 5 day treatment of urinary tract infection with various drugs in standard dosage

Drug	Cost*
Amoxycillin	£1.60
Cephalexin	£1.60
Co-trimoxazole	£1.26
Nalidixic acid	£3.54
Nitrofurantoin	6p
Oxytetracycline	13p
Sulphadimidine	12p

* Contract prices ruling at University College Hospital in July 1979. These prices will not be expected to apply elsewhere

generic name but by the brand name of the market leader, the cost would have been not 6p but approximately £1.50p.

For acute undifferentiated chest infection the clinical response will be similar with any of the following; amoxycillin, a cephalosporin, co-trimoxazole or oxytetracycline (or, indeed, with no antimicrobial agent). A 5 day course in standard dosage costs £1.60, £1.60, £1.26, 18p, respectively.

Clearly, in the light of such figures as these a policy can be constructed, according to the locally prevailing prices, which will save large sums of money without being detrimental to the wellbeing of patients. The main savings will be made not with the more spectacularly expensive but rarely prescribed drugs, but with the everyday drugs which are prescribed without much thought.

IMPLEMENTATION OF ANTIBIOTIC POLICIES

This subject has been well reviewed in Chapter 7 and elsewhere[5][6]. It is my belief that clinicians generally need, and welcome, advice from those more expert than themselves. In the United States of America this usually means communicable diseases specialists (physicians), in the United Kingdom it generally means clinical microbiologists, though some clinical pharmacologists or interested physicians undertake this work. What follows is an outline of the procedures followed at University College Hospital where the clinical microbiologists act as antibiotic advisers.

Our aim is to achieve all three objectives given above: (i) optimal patient treatment, (ii) control of antibiotic resistance, and (iii) low cost. We are a long way from complete success, but progress so far is encouraging.

Laboratory work
The first step is to provide as little laboratory encouragement to inappropriate prescribing as possible. When the clinical circumstances seem not to justify antibiotics, antibiotic sensitivity test results are not released, as in the case of intestinal pathogens from faecal samples, or the isolation of coliform organisms from varicose ulcers, for example. If the clinician asks why sensitivity results have not been given, we explain why we think chemotherapy is inappropriate. In addition, when a report on sensitivities is appropriate, the results released to the clinician are heavily censored in the laboratory so that only a few relatively safe, effective, 'clean', and cheap drugs are included. In the case of Group A *Streptococcus haemolyticus* or *Streptococcus pneumoniae*, for example, we

usually report only on penicillin. No more than four sensitivities are usually given for urinary pathogens. When an organism is mutliply resistant, full information is given. This means, for instance, that since cephalosporin sensitivities are rarely reported, this group of drugs is almost never used.

The next important step is to have a good network providing information. Careful record keeping of all pathogens isolated in the laboratory, complete with antibiotic sensitivities is important. We have a daily computer print-out of this, and a weekly computer analysis of all positive isolates by location. This gives us early warning of apparent cross-infection, or clustering of resistant strains which may repay attention. We receive information from the forms sent by clinicians requesting investigations on the nature of clinical problems and of any chemotherapy. The clinicians, or the medical students, or the nurses may mention problems arising on the wards.

Clinical work
Every day, members of the medical staff of the microbiology department do a ward round in the hospital. The first stop on this progress is at the Pharmacy, to collect a list of all the patients for whom antibiotics of any sort have been dispensed in the previous 24 hours. This list gives information on drug, dosage and route of administration. Anything unusual on that list occasions a visit to the patient. Any patient receiving aminoglycosides is visited in order to check that the drug is indicated, that dosage is appropriate and to arrange for assays to be done in the laboratory. Dosage is then adjusted by the microbiologists. Any patient receiving cephalosporins is visited, as are all patients receiving unusual dosages or on prolonged treatment with standard drugs.

Three areas are visited at least once a day, the intensive care unit, the premature baby unit and the paediatric unit. In these units particular care is taken to prevent the use of ecologically 'dirty' drugs such as ampicillin/amoxycillin. For lack of staff it is not yet possible for us to visit every patient receiving antibiotics, much though we should like to do so. Whenever possible we take microbiology trainees, technicians and medical students with us on our ward rounds. Exchanges of view with the clinicians at the bedside are routine, and offer an excellent opportunity for mutual education, and for instruction of medical students. We undertake some regular ward rounds with our clinical colleagues with recurring problems, such as the haematologists and oncologists looking after immunologically compromised patients, for instance.

Our approach is to support our clinical colleagues and offer constructive suggestions. We try to persuade our clinical colleagues who have mostly, over a period of time, learned to trust us. If we recommend changes in treatment we do so verbally to the clinical house staff and in writing in the patient's notes, while informing the nursing staff of our intentions. We do not give instructions, only advice which the clinicians may, but usually do not, reject.

How effective is this approach? In terms of obtaining the best clinical choice of drug we are aware of many instances of having helped the clinicians to help their patients. We are now asked for advice by the clinicians very much more often than formerly, which is taken as a vote of confidence. It must be admitted, however, that one or two units persist in what seem to us to be unsatisfactory antibiotic uses. In particular, the use of prophylactic chemotherapy in surgery is still, in my opinion, too great and somewhat irrational. In terms of protecting the environment, we have been modestly successful, mostly by preventing the use of some drugs in high dependency areas, and by achieving an overall reduction in antibiotic use. Table 1 shows that our big failure has been with amoxycillin/ampicillin, resistance to which is commoner now than previously, reflecting the great (too great) use of these drugs. On cost we have been very pleased with our efforts. In the last three years the cost of all drugs used at University College Hospital has more than doubled, yet the total sum spent on antimicrobial agents of all sorts has not increased at all. This can not be said of any other major group of drugs, but then no-one is attempting to control the use of other groups in quite the same sort of way. There is still no room for complacency, however, for examination of the use of chemotherapy at this hospital suggests to me that costs could still be reduced by three quarters without harm to patients. The saving in antibiotic costs achieved is of about the same size as the total cost of running the microbiology laboratory.

The key to the application of any policy of this sort is education, of microbiologists, laboratory technical staff, medical staff, medical students, nurses and pharmacists. Though much has been done, much more remains to be done. To be allowed to help in this work is enormous fun, and a great privilege.

References

1 Symmers, W. St.-C. (1973). Amphotericin Pharmacophobia. *Br. Med. J.*, **4**, 460
2 Price, D. J. E. and Sleigh, J. D. (1970). Control of infection due to *Klebsiella aerogenes* in a neurosurgical unit by withdrawal of all antibiotics. *Lancet*, **2**, 1213
3 Grüneberg, R. N. and Bendall, M. J. (1979). Hospital outbreak of trimethoprim resistance in pathogenic coliform bacteria. *Bri. Med. J.*, **2**, 7
4 Grüneberg, R. N., Smellie, J. M. and Leakey, A. (1973). Changes in the antibiotic sensitivities of faecal organisms in response to treatment in children with urinary tract infection. In *Urinary Tract Infection*, p. 131. W. Brumfitt and A. W. Asscher (eds.) (London: Oxford University Press)

5 Phillips, I. (1979). Antibiotic Policies. In D. S. Reeves and A. M. Geddes (eds.) *Recent Advances in Infection*, p. 151. (Edinburgh: Churchill Livingstone)
6 Lowbury, E. J. L., Ayliffe, G. A. J., Geddes, A. M. and Williams, J. D. (1975). *Control of Hospital Infection*, pp. 169–207. (London: Chapman and Hall)

Index

213